NO-RISK
Abs

A Safe Workout Program for Core Strength

Blandine Calais-Germain

Translated by Martine Curtis-Oakes

Healing Arts Press

Rochester, Vermont • Toronto, Canada

JESSAMINE COUNTY PUBLIC LIBRARY
600 South Main Street
Nicholasville, KY 40356
(859)885-3523

Healing Arts Press
One Park Street
Rochester, Vermont 05767
www.HealingArtsPress.com

Healing Arts Press is a division of Inner Traditions International

Copyright © 2008 by Éditions Désiris
English translation copyright © 2011 by Inner Traditions International

Originally published in French under the title *Abdos sans risque* by Éditions Désiris
First U.S. edition published in 2011 by Healing Arts Press

All rights reserved. No part of this book may be reproduced or utilized in any form or by any means, electronic or mechanical, including photocopying, recording, or by any information storage and retrieval system, without permission in writing from the publisher.

Note to the reader: This book is intended as an informational guide. The remedies, approaches, and techniques described herein are meant to supplement, and not to be a substitute for, professional medical care or treatment. They should not be used to treat a serious ailment without prior consultation with a qualified health care professional.

Library of Congress Cataloging-in-Publication Data

Calais-Germain, Blandine.
  [Abdos sans risque. English]
  No-risk abs : a safe workout program for core strength / Blandine Calais-Germain ; translated by Martine Curtis-Oakes.
     p. cm.
  Translated from French.
  Includes bibliographical references and index.
  ISBN 978-1-59477-389-1 (pbk.)
  1. Exercise. 2. Abdominal exercises. 3. Abdomen—Muscles. I. Title.
  GV508.C35 2011
  613.7'1—dc22

2010049224

Printed and bound in India by Replika Press Pvt. Ltd.

10 9 8 7 6 5 4 3 2

Drawings by Blandine Calais-Germain

Text design and layout by Virginia Scott Bowman
This book was typeset in Garamond Premier Pro with Helvetica Neue and Gill Sans as display typefaces

CONTENTS

PART ONE

What Are the Abs?

PART TWO

Abdominal Strength versus a Flat Belly

AUTHOR'S NOTE

This book invites you to understand, better evaluate, and mitigate the risks that are inherent in certain abdominal exercises. To get in shape, or stay in shape, we often look first to our midsections and decide that we're going to "work our abs." Exercises to strengthen and slim the midriff are featured in gyms, fitness clubs, and every magazine at grocery-store checkout counters.

But abdominal exercises are never without potential risk, because they place in motion the very core of our bodies, in which lie:

- The vertebral column
- The spinal cord
- The abdominal cavity and the perineum
- The organs of respiration, circulation, and digestion

All of these vital structures and systems can be damaged by the wrong exercises. Conversely, they can be protected by the appropriate kind of abdominal work.

No-Risk Abs lets you explore this poorly understood region of the body. Together we'll evaluate the most frequently recommended abdominal exercises, and then we'll see how we can improve on them. We'll explore:

- The risks associated with abdominal work
- The anatomical structures that make up the abs
- How to get "great abs"

No-Risk Abs is written not exclusively for medical professionals but also for anyone who wants to better understand, practice, or teach abdominal exercises. You'll find that the terminology in this book is designed to be accessible for the widest possible audience of readers. In particular, we have used the word *abs* to indicate the abdominal muscles in general, and/or the exercises that reinforce the trunk.

ACKNOWLEDGMENTS

For their invaluable help, the author would like to thank:

Antje Baumann

Anne Debreilly

Enrique Bruguera

Françoise Contreras

Stéphane Fernandes

Brigitte Hap

Christiane Mangiapani

Nuria Vives

PART ONE

· · · · · · · · · · · · · · · · · ·

What Are the Abs?

INTRODUCTION

It All Starts with the Abdominals

At birth, the newborn forcefully contracts his abdominals to push out the cry that signals his arrival into the world. And it was his mother's superhuman abdominal contractions that propelled the infant into this realm just moments earlier.

Those very same abdominal muscles are involved with every emotion we feel. We contract them when we cry, when we're angry, and when we're afraid. They're there every time we speak, and with every breath we take. As they relax and contract, they influence the movement and health of our organs. They initiate or follow the movements of our torso. They also stabilize the trunk to allow more range of motion for our arms and legs.

The Gym Isn't the Only Place to Work Your Abdominals

Almost every activity works the abdominals to some degree. For example . . .

- Singing or public speaking demands intense abdominal work, as the abdominals must constantly vary their force in order for the voice to achieve range and intensity.
- Movement practices such as tai chi and qigong require a constant play of the limbs in a standing position. The abdominals are active here not just to keep the trunk vertical but also, and perhaps even more importantly, to hold the organs in place.
- Holding the myriad yoga positions calls for abdominal support.
- Doing a session of push-ups requires the abdominals to stabilize the trunk and prevent the belly from pooching.

2

- Dancing calls on the abdominals to fix or mobilize the pelvis.
- Even in a period of relaxation, when the abdominals don't actively contract, abdominal work takes place. You must know the nature of "decontraction" to know the contracted state.

The Abdominals and Abdomen

The Abdominals

The abdominals are a group of four pairs of flat muscles that wrap a portion of the abdomen (the belly).

The first is the rectus abdominis, found at the front of the belly. (This is the muscle that yields what's commonly called "six-pack" abs.)

The other three, found on each side of the waist, are the transversus abdominis and the internal and external obliques. Together they form an overlapping muscle sheath three layers deep.

Working the Abs

"Working the abs" means performing exercises that reinforce the abdominal muscles.

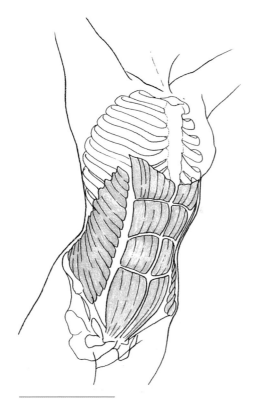

You can see that the abdominals form something like a chef's apron that wraps the front and sides of the trunk.

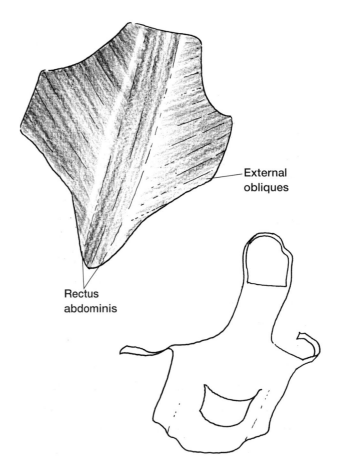

External obliques

Rectus abdominis

The Abdomen

The abdomen is the area that houses the viscera found below the diaphragm in the abdominal cavity. Above the diaphragm is the thoracic cavity.

The Abdominals
Play a Double Role

1 • *The Skeletal Role*

The abdominal muscles attach to several bones of the trunk: the ribs, the sternum, the vertebrae, and the pelvis. They can therefore mobilize these bones. This is their skeletal role.

For example, we can see below how the abdominals bring the trunk into flexion, moving the pelvis closer to the sternum.

2 • *The Visceral Role*

The abdominals make up a part of the envelope that encases the viscera of the abdomen, known as the abdominal sheath. When the abdominals contract, they can move the viscera, hold the viscera in place, or change their shape—a bit like a toothpaste tube. This is their visceral role.

For example, here we see how the abdominals can pull the belly in without any movement of the trunk.

These two roles, skeletal and visceral, are often in play at the same time during a movement, making it difficult to analyze the movement's effects. For this reason, in the exercises in this book we will always indicate whether the role of the abdominals is skeletal or visceral.

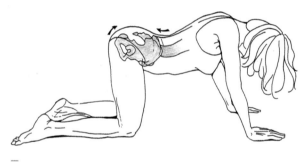

Without abdominals

1

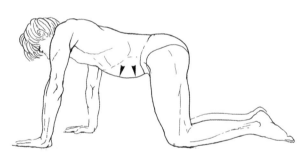

Without abdominals

2

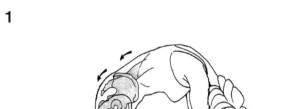

With abdominals

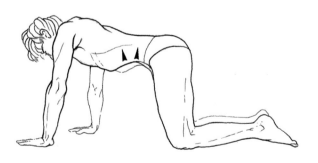

With abdominals

The Abdominal Cavity

The abdominal cavity is the entirety of the "container" that holds the viscera of the abdomen. Though it's often wrongly thought to be just the abdominal muscles, this cavity is made up of bony regions as well as muscles.

The word *container* isn't quite accurate, as it brings to mind something rigid, like a box. The abdominal cavity is in fact very flexible—and flexible in every direction—not just because it's made up in part of muscles, but because the bones that help make it up contain many joints:

- There are the joints between the vertebrae
- There are numerous joints in the rib cage

In addition, the ribs themselves, which are intricately related to the abs, can open or close to some degree, especially the lower ribs.

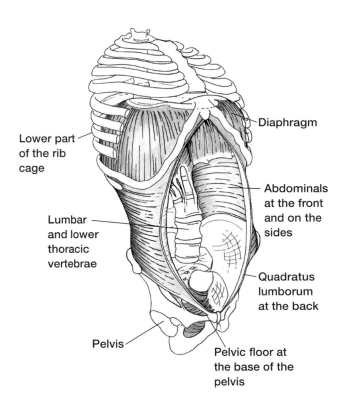

The abdominal cavity is a flexible container.

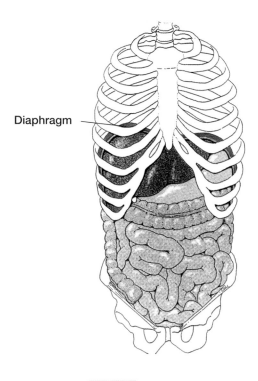

The abdomen houses the viscera below the diaphragm.

THE RECTUS ABDOMINIS

Locating the Rectus Abdominis

Description

There are two rectus abdominis muscles, one on each side of the midline of the belly. Among the abdominal muscles, these are the only ones that are found at the front. They form the only muscle layer at the front of the belly.

The rectus abdominis muscles have an easily recognizable form: the contractile fibers (reddish) are broken by noncontractile zones (whitish). This structure gives the muscles their "six-pack" form.

Insertion

At the top, each rectus abdominis muscle attaches on either side of the sternum at the cartilage of the fifth, sixth, and seventh ribs. They narrow as they descend almost directly down the front of the belly and attach to the front of the pelvis at the pubis.

The rectus abdominis muscles extend vertically along the entire length of the belly.

How the Rectus Abdominis Acts on the Skeleton

1 • *Retroversion*

The rectus abdominis can pull on the pelvis, bringing the pubis toward the sternum and eliminating the arch of the lower back (the lower back rounds and the buttocks tuck under). This tucking of the pelvis is called retroversion. The rectus abdominis also prevent the pelvis from moving in the opposite direction.

2 • *Dropping the Ribs*

The rectus abdominis can pull the sternum and the front of the rib cage toward the pelvis, which causes the ribs to drop. It can fix the ribs in this dropped position and also prevent them from lifting. (Note that when we drop the ribs in this fashion, we tend to exhale.)

3 • *Flexion of the Spine*

Indirectly, by pulling on the pelvis or the ribs, the rectus abdominis can cause flexion (rounding) of the spine. It can also inhibit the spine's movement in the opposite direction (for example, it prevents arching the back).

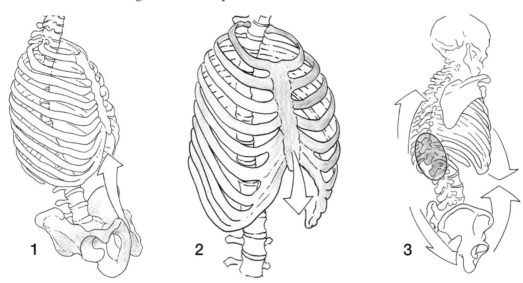

Important Note

We need to note three things here:

- The rectus abdominis does not act directly on the spine because it isn't attached to any vertebrae.
- By acting on the lower thoracic rib cage and the pelvis, the rectus abdominis affects the lower thoracic vertebrae, the lumbar vertebrae, and the lumbothoracic and lumbosacral "hinges."
- Of these affected regions, the most mobile is the lumbothoracic hinge—where the twelfth thoracic vertebra meets the first lumbar vertebra. As a result, the rectus abdominis has greatest effect in this area; it tends to round the midback (in the region of the lower ribs) more than it reduces the curve of the lower back (in the lumbar region). If we want it to flatten the lumbar curve, we first need to inhibit flexion in the midback.

How the Rectus Abdominis Acts on the Viscera

When contracted, the rectus abdominis pushes the viscera backward, moving them closer to the spine.

Important Note

When pushed, the viscera don't decrease in volume. This is impossible, as they are like a volume of incompressible liquid. Instead the viscera change form, compacting out to the sides of the abdomen, up toward the thorax, and down toward the pelvis.

The rectus abdominis rarely contracts along its entire length; instead, it contracts region by region. For example, it can contract uniquely below the ribs, at the level of the navel, or above the pelvis.

The rectus abdominis's ability to move the belly by successively contracting at different levels means that it can move the viscera toward either the thorax or the pelvis.

The rectus abdominis is the director-in-chief of the belly, which it can move upward or downward. Its action is often coupled with the action of other abdominal muscles, but it's the action of the rectus that most profoundly influences the movement of the belly.

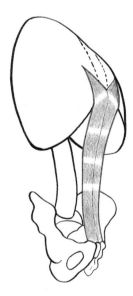

Fully contracted rectus abdominis

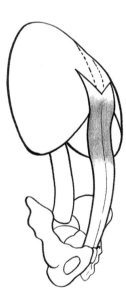

Contraction below the ribs

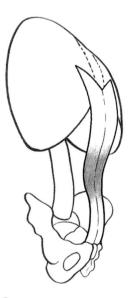

Contraction at the level of the navel

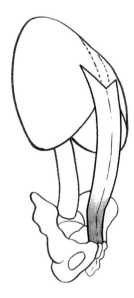

Contraction above the pelvis

THE BROAD MUSCLES AND THE ABDOMINAL APONEUROSES

✦ **The Broad Muscles**

✦ **The Aponeuroses of the Abdominals**

The Broad Muscles

The abdominals found on the sides of the body are called the broad muscles (as opposed to the elongated form of the rectus abdominis in the front). There are three broad muscles on each side, superimposed in three layers and covering each other almost completely.

From the deepest to the most superficial, they are:

- The transversus abdominis
- The internal oblique
- The external oblique

This triple layer of muscles can be quite thin in slight people. Conversely, it can be more developed and extend beyond the bony limits of the pelvis in very muscular people. (Of course, it can also increase in size with weight gain, but that has nothing to do with muscle.)

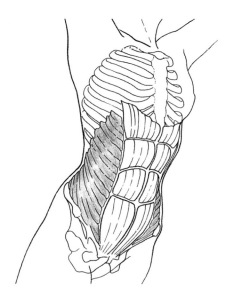

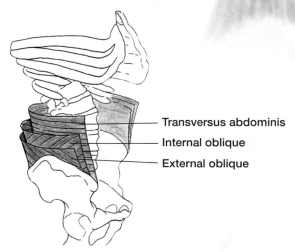

Transversus abdominis

Internal oblique

External oblique

The Aponeuroses of the Abdominals

Look at any muscle and you will see areas of red and white. This is true for the abdominals as well. Like all muscles, they are composed of two types of fibers:

- Contractile fibers (the red areas), the "active" part of the muscle
- Aponeuroses (the white areas), which do not contract

Aponeuroses can take two forms, each with its own function:

- They can envelop the muscle like a sheath.
- They can form flat, fibrous sheets of connective tissue that extend the contractile reach of muscles. In the abdominals, these extensions are found at the front of the belly and are called the anterior aponeuroses.

The Anterior Aponeuroses of the Broad Muscles

Each of the three broad muscles is enveloped in two aponeuroses, one deep and one superficial. There are therefore six aponeuroses in all, and they overlap one another, separating and fusing to envelop the rectus abdominis before rejoining at the midline of the body to form the linea alba. This rather complex arrangement varies according to the level:

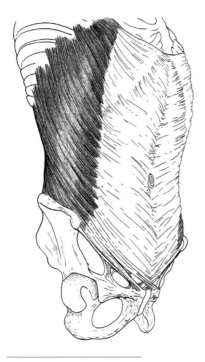

The external obliques and their aponeuroses

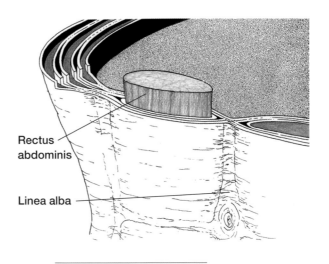

Rectus abdominis

Linea alba

The aponeuroses of the broad muscles envelop the rectus abdominis and join at the linea alba.

- In the upper two-thirds of the abdomen, the aponeuroses of the transversus abdominis and the deep aponeurosis of the internal oblique pass behind the rectus abdominis. Simultaneously, the aponeuroses of the external oblique and the superficial aponeurosis of the internal oblique pass in front of the rectus abdominis.
- In the lower one-third of the abdomen, all the aponeuroses of the broad muscles pass in front of the rectus abdominis. This area is visible in the lower abdomen where it forms a horizontal line, below which the belly looks a bit more pulled in.

The Linea Alba

All of the connective tissues coming from the broad muscles on the sides of the abdomen (the aponeuroses) come together and commingle their fibers to form what is called the linea alba or "white line." This intersection of fibers makes for an area of strength. Yet the linea alba also has several points of weakness where hernias can develop. (See "Hernia of the Linea Alba" on page 34.)

THE TRANSVERSUS ABDOMINIS

+ Locating the Transversus Abdominis
+ How the Transversus Abdominis Acts on the Skeleton
+ How the Transversus Abdominis Acts on the Viscera

Locating the Transversus Abdominis

Description

There are two transversus abdominis muscles, one on each side of the body. Of the three broad muscles found on the sides of the waist, the transversus abdominis is the deepest. It is practically up against the organs and viscera, separated from them by only a layer of fascia. The transversus abdominis is covered by the other two layers of abdominal muscles.

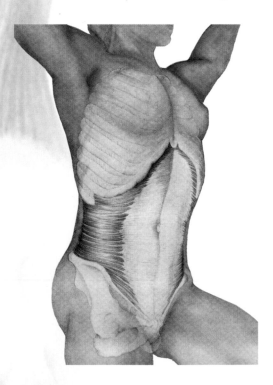

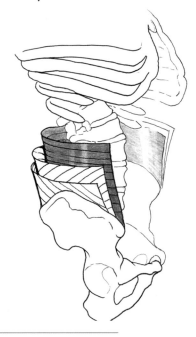

The contractile (red) fibers of the transversus abdominis run horizontally at the sides of the waist.

12

Insertion

At its upper end, the transversus abdominis attaches to the inferior surface of the thoracic rib cage. At its bottom, it attaches to the iliac crest of the pelvis, at the spot where you would place your hands on your hips, and extends along the inguinal ligament of the groin.

At the front of the abdomen, the fibers of the transversus abdominis on each side come together via the anterior aponeuroses. Recall that the muscle has two aponeuroses, one deep (seen in the drawing) and one superficial. These two aponeuroses pass in front of the rectus abdominis in the lower third of the belly but behind the rectus abdominis in the upper two-thirds of the belly.

How the Transversus Abdominis Acts on the Skeleton

The transversus abdominis can't pull on the pelvis because its contractile fibers run parallel to the pelvis.

The muscle doesn't mobilize the vertebrae. Or at least it doesn't do so more than just barely; the circular tightening of the transversus abdominis around the waist could possibly pull on the lumbar vertebrae and deepen the lumbar curve. But this presupposes that the anterior (front) portion of the muscle is fixed, and this action is therefore more true in theory than in reality.

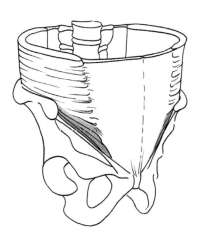

The transverse abdominis extending along the inguinal ligament

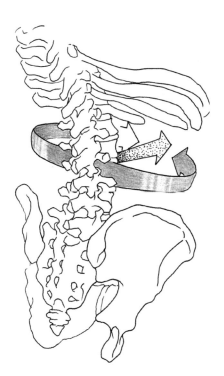

The transversus abdominis can pull the ribs closer together at the front of the body. However, this action is minimal because the muscle's fibers between the ribs are very short.

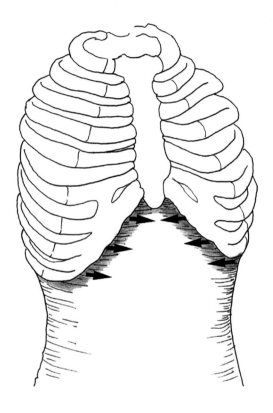

How the Transversus Abdominis Acts on the Viscera

The transverse abdominal muscle acts on two regions of the belly in particular.

1 • Narrowing the Waist

The transversus abdominis performs a significant action in the area between the ribs and the pelvis, where its fibers are the longest and

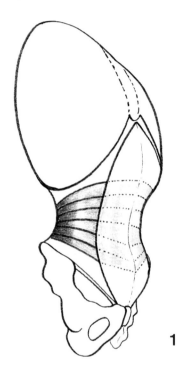

1

The transversus abdominis has almost no action on the skeleton. Of all of the abdominal muscles, it acts the least on the skeleton. Its action is primarily on the viscera.

the most numerous. When contracted, it narrows the waist, pushing the viscera up toward the thorax or down toward the pelvis. (When we're standing, they most often move downward, as gravity is already pulling them in that direction.)

However, the transversus adominis's ability to direct the viscera toward the pelvis or the thorax is weak, which is why its action needs to be completed by the action of the other abdominals:

- The rectus abdominis pushing the viscera up or down
- The internal obliques pulling in the upper part of the belly and therefore pushing the viscera down
- The external obliques pulling in the lower belly and therefore pushing the viscera up

The transversus abdominis is more the muscle of the "narrow waist" than the "flat belly."

2 • Supporting the Lower Abdomen

The transversus abdominis has a very specific and subtle action at its lower end, where its fibers run along the inguinal ligament to a point about midway along the ligament. When contracted, the muscle helps support the lower abdomen, complementing the action of the internal oblique.

The transversus abdominis can be contracted region by region.

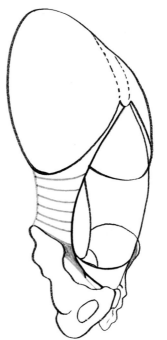

2

THE INTERNAL OBLIQUES

Locating the Internal Obliques

Description

There is an internal oblique muscle on each side of the abdomen. Of the three broad muscles found on the sides of the waist, the internal obliques form the middle layer. They are situated under the external obliques and on top of the tranversus abdominis muscles.

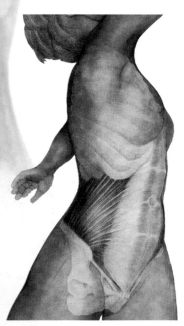

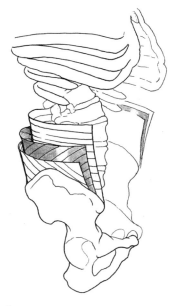

The contractile (red) fibers of the internal obliques wrap the sides of the waist as they ascend from the pelvis to the rib cage.

Insertion

At its top, the internal oblique muscle attaches to the edge of the thoracic rib cage. At its bottom, it attaches to the iliac crest of the pelvis (the spot where you would put your hand

16

on your hip) and extends along the inguinal ligament of the groin. At this lower level, the internal obliques have the longest and most significant fibers of all the broad muscles.

At the front of the abdomen, the aponeuroses of the right and left internal obliques meet at the linea alba, at the midline of the belly.

How the Internal Obliques Act on the Skeleton

1 • *Side Bending and Forward Pelvic Rotation*

An internal oblique can pull on the pelvis.

- It can pull the pelvis laterally toward the ribs (lateral inclination or side bending), and it can inhibit the movement of the pelvis in the opposite direction.
- It can rotate the pelvis forward, and it can inhibit its rotation in the opposite direction.

2 • *Flattening the Rib Cage*

An internal oblique can pull the front of the rib cage downward and toward the side of the pelvis, and it can inhibit its return to the starting position. The rib cage gets flatter and wider in this movement. (Note that when we drop the ribs like this we tend to exhale.)

3 • *Indirectly Mobilizing the Vertebrae*

By pulling the pelvis or rib cage laterally (to the side), an internal oblique can indirectly mobilize certain vertebrae, bending or rotating the spine at the waist, and inhibiting the spine's movement in the opposite direction. It isn't directly responsible for moving the spine, as it doesn't attach to any vertebrae.

Situated obliquely at the sides of the trunk, the fibers of the internal obliques mobilize the sides on which they contract.

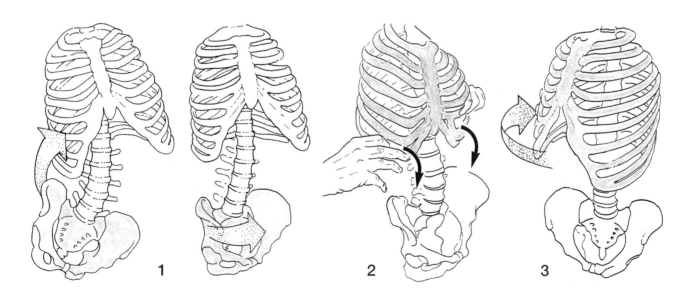

How the Internal Obliques Act on the Viscera

The internal obliques act in two particular regions of the belly.

1 • Compressing the Viscera above the Navel

The internal obliques exert a major action at their upper end (where the longest fibers terminate): when contracted, they press on the viscera principally above the navel, pushing them down toward the pelvis or out to the sides.

2 • Supporting the Lower Abdomen

The internal obliques have a specific and subtle action at their lower end, along the inguinal ligament, where their lower fibers are longest and most significant: when contracted, the muscles reinforce the inguinal ligament and contribute to supporting the lower abdomen.

The internal obliques can contract region by region. For example, they can contract strictly above the navel, at the level of the navel, or at the lower level where they border the pelvis. This means that we can pull in our belly in stages.

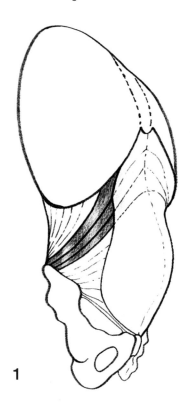

1

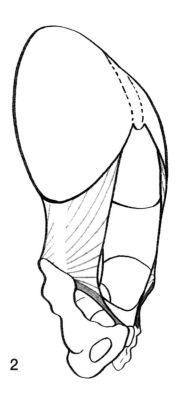

2

The internal obliques act on the viscera by tightening the belly, primarily in the area above the navel. They often act in conjunction with other abdominals.

THE EXTERNAL OBLIQUES

- ✦ Locating the External Obliques
- ✦ How the External Obliques Act on the Skeleton
- ✦ How the External Obliques Act on the Viscera

Locating the External Obliques

Description

There is an external oblique muscle on each side of the abdomen. Of the three broad muscles found on the sides of the waist, the external obliques are the most superficial. They are found just under the skin, and the internal oblique and transversus abdominis muscles lie beneath them.

Insertion

At their upper ends, the external obliques attach primarily to the sides and front of the

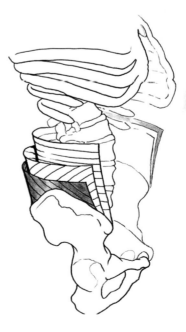

The contractile (red) fibers of the external obliques wrap the sides of the waist as they descend from the ribs to the pelvis.

rib cage. At their lower ends, they attach to the iliac crest of the pelvis (where you would put your hands on your hips). They extend, by way of tendinous fibers, along the inguinal ligament of the groin.

At the front of the abdomen, the aponeuroses of the right and left external obliques meet at the linea alba.

How the External Obliques Act on the Skeleton

1 • *Side Bending and Backward Pelvic Rotation*

An external oblique can pull on the pelvis.

- It can pull the pelvis laterally toward the ribs (lateral inclination or side bending), and it can inhibit the movement of the pelvis in the opposite direction.
- It can rotate the pelvis backward, and it can inhibit its rotation in the opposite direction.

2 • *Narrowing the Rib Cage*

An external oblique can pull the thoracic ribs down toward the middle of the trunk, and it can inhibit their return to the starting position. The rib cage narrows in this movement. (Note that when we drop our rib cage like this, we tend to exhale.) If the rib cage doesn't change its shape, the external oblique will cause it to turn to the front.

3 • *Indirectly Mobilizing the Vertebrae*

By pulling the pelvis or rib cage laterally (to the side), an external oblique can indirectly mobilize certain vertebrae, bending or rotating the spine at the waist, and inhibiting the spine's movement in the opposite direction. It isn't directly responsible for moving the spine, as it doesn't attach to any of the vertebrae.

Situated obliquely on the sides of the trunk, the fibers of the external obliques mobilize the sides on which they contract.

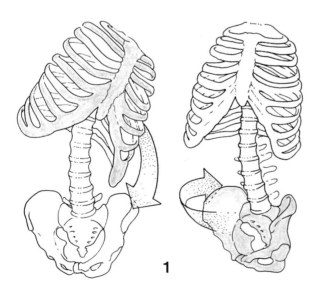

1

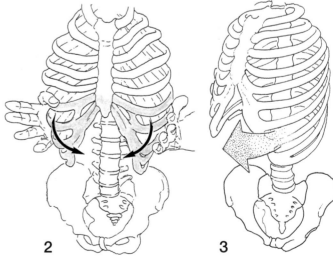

2   3

How the External Obliques Act on the Viscera

The external obliques act in two specific regions of the belly.

1 • *Compressing the Viscera below the Navel*

The external obliques have a significant impact in the area of the lower belly, where their fibers are the longest: upon contraction, they press on the viscera principally below the navel, pushing them up toward the ribs. In addition, contraction of the external oblique on one side can push the viscera to the opposite side; it can move the viscera laterally.

2 • *Supporting the Lower Abdomen*

The external obliques have a specific action at their lower end: Their fibers stretch from the ninth and tenth ribs to the inguinal ligament, which is sometimes considered the tendon of the external oblique. When these fibers contract, the action pulls on the inguinal ligament and contributes to supporting the lower abdomen.

The external obliques can contract zone by zone. For example, they can contract at the level of the waist or at the level of the ribs. This means that we can pull in our belly in stages.

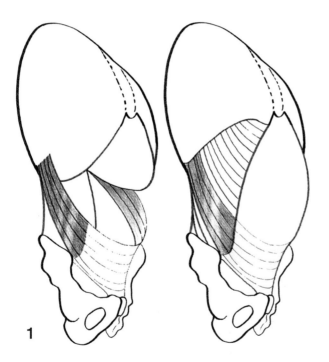

1

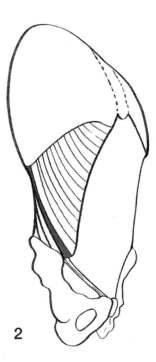

2

The external obliques can push the viscera up toward the thorax or out to the sides. They often act in conjunction with other abdominals.

UNDERSTANDING SOME KEY WORDS

The Pelvis and the Inguinal Ligament

The pelvis is formed by an ensemble of four bones at the base of the trunk and has a flared form. We can feel the top of the pelvis when we put our hands on the hips; these points are called the iliac crests. The most forward part of the iliac crest is a protrusion called the anterior superior iliac spine (ASIS). The pubic bone or pubis, where the two iliac bones are joined by a layer of fibrocartilage, lies below and in front of the iliac bones.

The Pelvis and the Abdominals
The abdominal muscles attach to certain parts of the iliac bones but not to the sacrum or the coccyx.

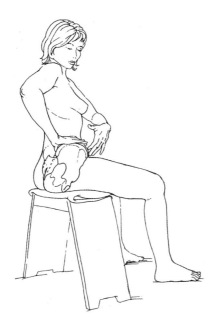

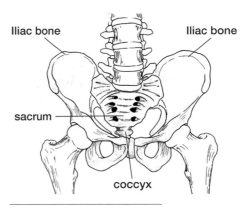

The four bones of the pelvis

- The transversus abdominis muscles, the external obliques, and the internal obliques (the broad muscles) attach to the iliac crest.
- The rectus abdominis muscles attach to the pubic bone.

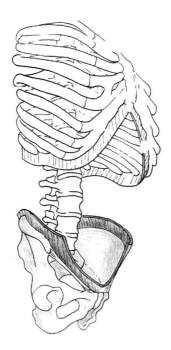

The Inguinal Ligament

The inguinal ligament is a fibrous cord, sometimes called the crural arch, that runs from the anterior superior iliac spine (ASIS) to the top of the pubic bone. The abdominal broad muscles attach to and help support the inguinal ligament. The contractile fibers of the transversus abdominis run to the middle of the inguinal ligament. The contractile fibers of the internal oblique run further along the ligament to the pubic bone, and in men they continue to the scrotum, forming the cremaster muscle. The contractile fibers of the external oblique terminate at the ASIS. The inguinal ligament is considered to be the terminal point of contractile fibers coming from the ninth and tenth ribs, almost as if it were the tendon of these fibers.

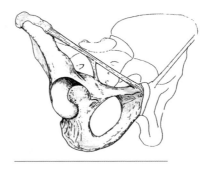

The inguinal ligament

How the Abdominals Move the Pelvis

The abdominal muscles directly initiate certain movements of the pelvis.

1 • *Retroversion*

The abdominals can initiate retroversion, or the tucking under of the pelvis. This movement takes the iliac crest backward, so that the ASIS tips back and up. It is often associated with flattening out the lumbar spine. The rectus abdominis is the retroverter.

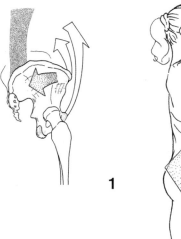

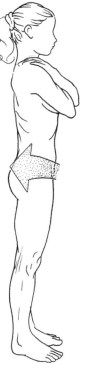

2 • *Lateral Inclination*

The abdominals can also initiate lateral inclination of the pelvis, pivoting it from side to side. The obliques play a dominant role in this movement.

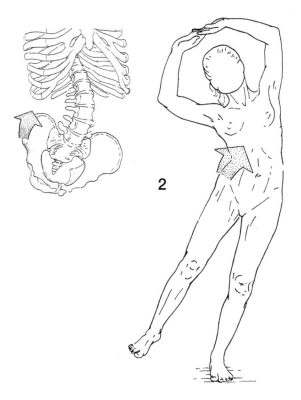

3 • *Rotation*

The abdominals can rotate the pelvis, turning it clockwise or counterclockwise. The obliques are the actors in pelvic rotation.

One pelvic movement that the abdominals are not responsible for is anteversion, which takes the iliac crest forward, advancing the ASIS. Anteversion of the pelvis is often associated with aching of the lumbar spine and lordosis. The abdominals (primarily the rectus abdominis)

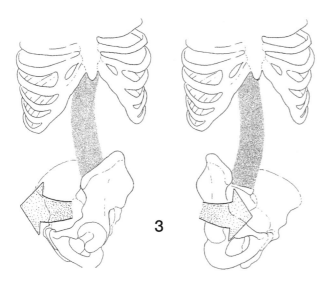

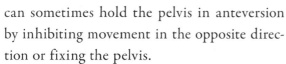

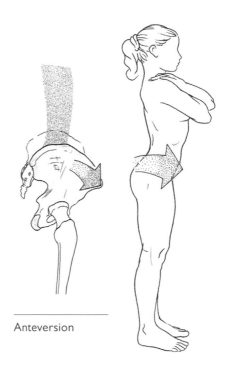

Anteversion

can sometimes hold the pelvis in anteversion by inhibiting movement in the opposite direction or fixing the pelvis.

The Spine and the Lumbar Spine

The Spine

The central axis of the skeletal system, the spine is composed of twenty-four vertebrae, the

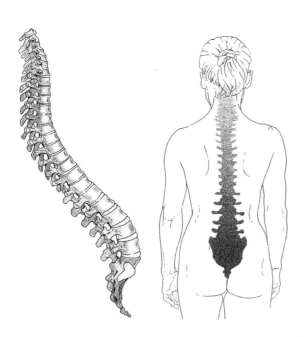

sacrum, and the coccyx. It contains the spinal cord and nerve roots and is connected to three structures: the head, the rib cage, and the pelvis. When seen in profile, it forms three curves.

With its seventy-four joints and twenty-three intervertebral disks, the spine is very articulated. It can become a rigid and solid pillar of support for the trunk or, alternately, a flexible and mobile link, courtesy of the numerous muscles that can stabilize or move it.

The abdominal muscles serve to either stabilize and fix the spine or, conversely, to mobilize it. The abdominals act on both the thoracic and the lumbar vertebrae. Their action, however, is never direct, as these muscles don't attach directly to the spine. Their effect on the spine comes, instead, through their action on the pelvis or the rib cage.

The Lumbar Spine

The lumbar spine is that part of the spine that occurs at waist level, between the ribs and the

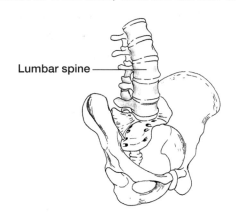

Lumbar spine

pelvis. It's a region where the vertebrae are at once massive (because they are the lowest vertebrae) and, at the same time, mobile (because they have no ribs attached to them).

The lumbar spine bears the greatest load of all the vertebrae, and for this reason we often feel pain here, in particular in two regions: between L5 (the lowest lumbar vertebra) and the sacrum, and between L4 and L5. Pain in this area may arise from the intervertebral disks (compressed or herniated), from the nerves that pass through the spine at this level (particularly the sciatic nerve), or from the ligaments and muscles that hold the vertebrae together.

Movements of the Lumbar and Lower Thoracic Spine

1 • Extension

Bending the lumbar spine backward is called extension, or lordosis. The role of the abdominals is to inhibit this movement, as necessary. The spine is very mobile in extension at its lowest levels (L5/S1, L4/L5).

2 • Flexion

Bending the lumbar spine forward is called flexion, and it causes a flattening of the lower back. Flexion is limited in the lumbar area but becomes

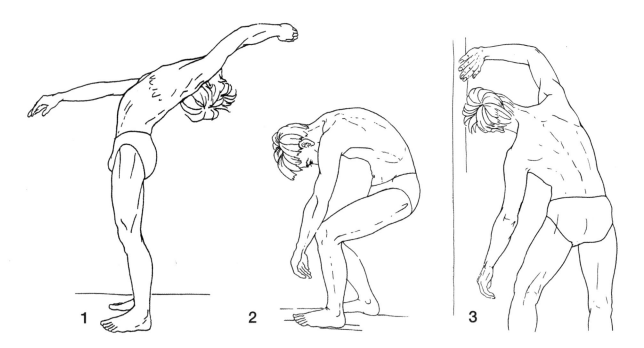

1   2   3

more and more possible as we move up the spine. The spine is has significant mobility in flexion in the upper lumbar (L1) and lower thoracic (T11, T12) spine. It's this area—the lumbothoracic hinge—that tends to bend first under the action of the abdominals.

3 • Lateral Inclination

Bending the lumbar spine to the side is called lateral flexion or lateral inclination. The spine has greatest mobility in lateral flexion in the lumbar spine; higher up the spine, the side-bending movement is restricted by the ribs. However, lateral flexion does not involve the lowest two vertebrae of the spine, because ligaments restrict them from bending in this direction.

4 • Rotation

Turning the spine to the side is called rotation, and it is just barely possible in the lumbar region because of the form the vertebrae take here. Rotation really starts to happen at T11 and T12, at the bottom of the rib cage.

The lower levels of the lumbar spine are very mobile in extension. In flexion, the spine has maximal movement at the lumbothoracic level (T11–L1). In lateral flexion, or lateral inclination, the spine has greatest mobility in the lumbar spine. Rotation, on the other hand, is barely possible at the level of the lumbar spine; it starts to happen at T11/T12.

The Intervertebral Disk

The intervertebral disk is a piece of fibrous cartilage that unites two vertebrae, or, more exactly, two vertebral bodies (the anterior parts of the vertebrae). The disk, which looks a bit like an onion slice, is made up of a slightly gelatinous nucleus surrounded by concentric rings of fibrocartilage.

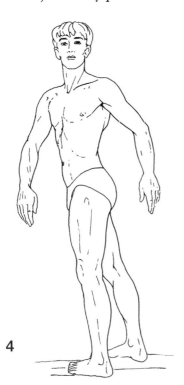

4

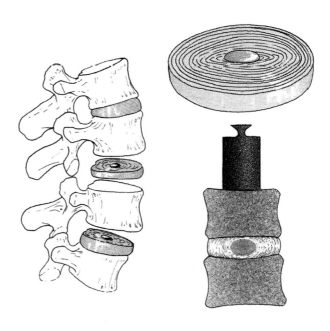

Important Note

The following exercises are high-pressure exercises that can put tremendous pressure on the intervertebral disks:

- Crunches, if they are done as complete roll-ups or with an arched back (see pages 66–70).
- Leg lifts, if the pelvis isn't stable (see page 78).
- Torsion of the trunk (see page 86).

Intervertebral disks allow movement between the vertebrae and cushion the weight put on the spine when we move our trunk and limbs. Though their load-bearing capacity increases as we travel down the spine, the disks are fragile and need to be protected. They don't repair themselves when they are damaged. We need to avoid overtaxing them, especially the lumbar disks, as they are the ones that take most of the abuse, thanks to their load-bearing role.

When we do abdominal exercises, we must avoid putting unnecessary pressure on the intervertebral disks, especially when we're making movements that tend to compress them.

The Dorsals

The dorsals are a group of back muscles, or, more exactly, the muscles situated along the spine (the deepest; see illustration 1), the muscles at the back of the ribs (not quite as deep), and the latissimus dorsi, a broad muscle that runs from the pelvis to the arm (the most superficial; see illustration 2).

As a group, these muscles cause the opposite action of the abdominals:

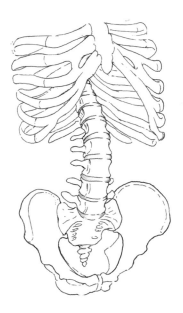

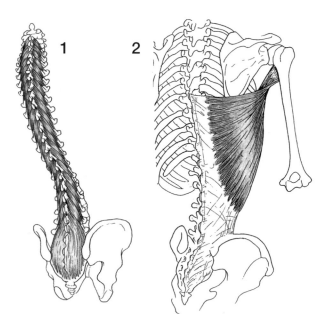

- Most antevert the pelvis.
- They extend the spine (arching the back), causing the ribs to rise in the front.

The Importance of Spinal Lordosis

The spine has a slight natural arch in the lower back, what we call a physiological lordosis. When working the abdominals, it's necessary to keep this natural lordotic curve whenever possible. That is to say, we try to keep the natural curve of the spine even though the abdominals tend to flatten it out.

Working in this natural position of the spine lets us integrate the abdominals optimally, rather than in a position that causes the spine and the rib cage to collapse. It's especially important to maintain this position when we recruit the abdominals on a strong exhalation (for example, when we play a wind instrument for an extended time).

The Abdominals and Dorsals Stabilize the Pelvis

In certain exercises where we lift and lower our legs (see pages 75–79), it's necessary to stabilize the pelvis to avoid going into anteversion (the job of the abdominals) or retroversion (the job of the dorsals). So the abdominals and dorsals work in conjunction here, either alternating or simultaneously.

Whenever possible, work the abdominals and the dorsals (back muscles) at the same time to maintain a lordotic curve of the lower spine. Certain exercises recruit both muscle groups to stabilize the pelvis.

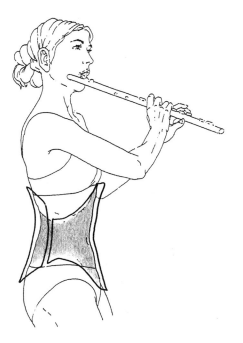

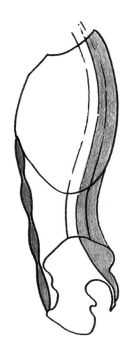

The Rib Cage

The rib cage is the skeleton of the thorax and forms the top of the abdomen. It is made up of twelve pairs of ribs, bones that are at the same time flat and curved.

At the front of the body, the rib cage contains costal cartilage (cartilage coming from the ribs), with the sternum right in the middle.

At the back of the body, the rib cage includes the thoracic spine, which is composed of twelve thoracic vertebrae and their joints.

The rib cage is a very mobile unit, and when we work the abdominals, we sometimes need to move it and at other times need to stabilize it.

Unlike the pelvis, the rib cage is not rigid: when the abdominals pull on the ribs, they tend to close the rib cage. When we're doing abdominal exercises, we sometimes try to hold the rib cage like a solid block in its expanded state. Maintaining this position is a function of the intercostal muscles, the inspiratory muscles of the rib cage.

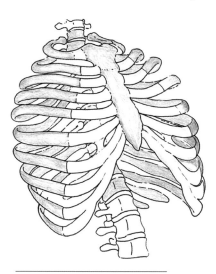

Front of the rib cage

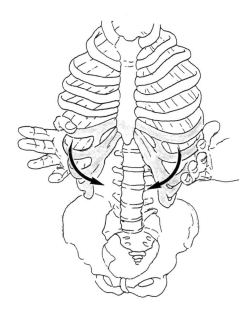

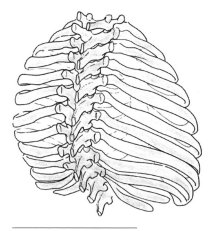

Back of the rib cage

The abdominals always pull the rib cage downward.

When the rib cage descends:
- We tend to exhale; the abdominals are therefore muscles of exhalation.
- We tend to flex our spine.
- We tend to pull in our abdomen, pushing it toward the pelvis.

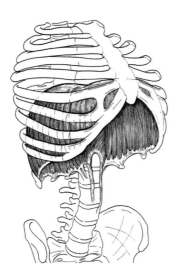
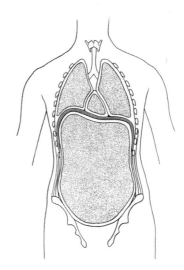

The Diaphragm

The diaphragm is a thin and supple cupola-shaped muscle situated between the thorax and the abdomen. It attaches to the inside of the rib cage.

The diaphragm is, above all, the principal muscle of inhalation. When it contracts, it descends, pulling with it the lungs, which then enlarge downward. This pulls air into the lungs, or, in other words, we inhale. The contraction of the diaphragm pushes the belly toward the pelvis (downward), and the belly expands.

With this type of inhalation, the action of the diaphragm opposes that of the transversus abdominis: the diaphragm contracts while the transversus abdominis relaxes. This is the best-known kind of diaphragmatic breathing, and we often call it belly breathing.

However, the abdominals can remain tonic

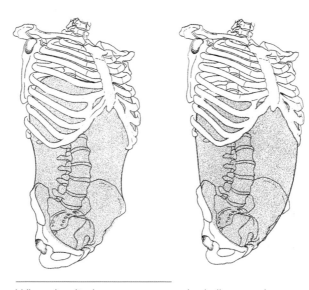

When the diaphragm contracts, the belly expands.

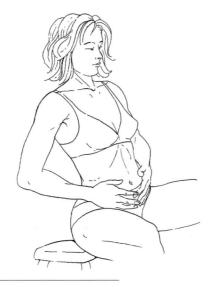

(partially contracted) when the diaphragm contracts. In this case the diaphragm can't descend entirely, and the abdomen remains fixed. This causes the ribs to flare and move upward; the belly does not expand. For the diaphragm to react in this way, it's necessary to keep some tonus (contraction) in the abdominals.

> The interplay between the diaphragm and the abdominals is changeable. What's important to remember is that these muscles work in coordination.

Diaphramatic, or belly, breathing

The Glottis

The glottis is the space between the vocal cords, which stretch to the inside of the thyroid cartilage (better known as the Adam's apple).

The vocal cords can be separated (when we breathe), brought together (to form sounds), or squeezed together tightly when we absolutely have to restrict the airflow (for example, right before we cough or when we hiccup).

In the course of doing intense abdominal exercise, we tend to close the glottis tightly while continuing to "push" air against it (sometimes called a glottal stop or *coup de glotte*).

This allows us to keep the thorax open during the effort. However, the pressure against the glottis builds and is directed in the opposite direction, downward toward the abdomen or the perineum.

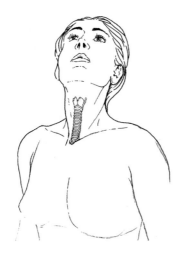

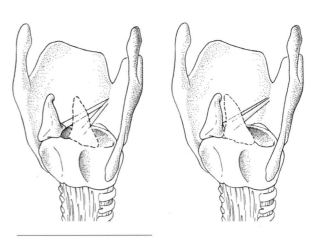

The vocal cords can be separated or closed.

Hernias

A hernia is a condition in which an organ protrudes through the tissues that contain it. Hernias are common in the abdominal region, which often is under pressure and requires resistance from the abdominal walls. Hernias appear in weak spots in the abdominal wall. When it happens at the level of the perineum, a hernia is called a prolapse.

Femoral Hernia

At their lower end, the abdominals attach to the inguinal ligament. Just below the inguinal ligament is the femoral canal, through which vital elements pass from the trunk to the leg: the femoral vein, the femoral artery, and the femoral nerve. Midway along the inguinal ligament, a small ligament runs back to the pelvis, anchoring the inguinal ligament more strongly to the pelvis. The femoral canal is a breach through which the small intestines can sometimes protrude. This is called a femoral hernia.

Inguinal Hernia

The abdominals attach to the superior (upper) border of the inguinal ligament. At this level, in the area close to the pubic bone, there is a small slot: the inguinal ring, which serves as a passageway for elements running between the inside and outside of the pelvis:

- The spermatic cord in men, which attaches the testicles to the seminal vesicles
- The round ligament in women

The inguinal ring is formed where the broad muscles of the abdomen overlap, leaving a gap. The small intestine can protrude or even break through this breach in the abdominal cavity, resulting in an inguinal hernia.

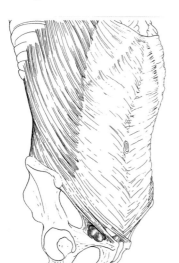

Femoral hernia

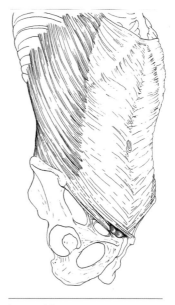

Inguinal hernia

Hernia of the Linea Alba

When the linea alba is distended, it can become thinner and, subsequently, weaker in spots, and it can even develop small fissures. A portion of the small intestine can protrude or even break through at a weakened point. This is called a hernia of the linea alba.

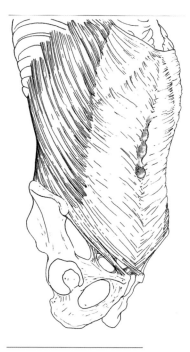

Hernia of the linea alba and umbilicus

Umbilical Hernia

When the linea alba is distended at the navel, this area weakens and can't easily withstand any pressure put on it. Instead of going inward, the belly button pokes out, and the small intestine can begin to protrude or pop out at this weakened point. This is what we call an umbilical hernia.

Any situation that increases pressure in the abdomen can aggravate a hernia.

Around the Perineum

The perineum is the found at the lowest level of the trunk. It's made up of a variety of tissues: skin, muscles, fat, erectile bodies, viscera (the bladder, and the uterus and vagina in females), ligaments, vessels, and nerves. The word *perineum* sometimes is used to designate all of these structures, while at other times it designates just the structures found between the lowest viscera and the skin.

The Pelvic Floor

The term *pelvic floor* designates specifically the muscles of the perineum. It includes all of the muscles in this area, from the superficial to the deep, and from the muscles of support that form the surface of the pelvic floor to the sphincter muscles that form the openings.

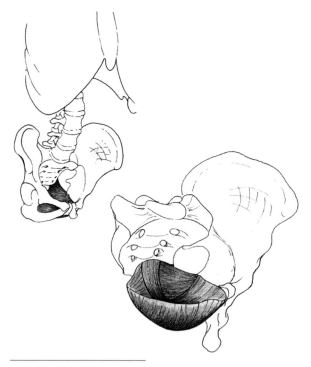

The pelvic floor

The Greater and Small Pelvis

The interior of the pelvis is divided into two levels. The upper region, which is also the widest, is called the greater pelvis or pelvis major. The narrower, lower area is the small pelvis or pelvis minor. The viscera of the perineum are located within the pelvis minor.*

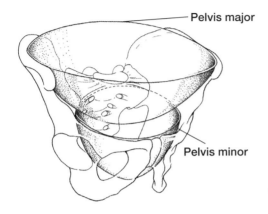

Pelvis major

Pelvis minor

Prolapse and Incontinence

Prolapse

Prolapse is the slipping or dropping down of an organ of the small pelvis out of its normal place. The three viscera of the small pelvis in females—the bladder, uterus, and vagina—are often subject to prolapse, which can be caused by deterioration of the ligaments or weakness of the muscles that support them.

Repeated pressure on the perineum can contribute to prolapse. Movement in daily life exposes the perineum to a multitude of pressures. This is why it is doubly important to avoid adding more pressure on the region while doing abdominal exercises.

*For more details on the perineum, see *The Female Pelvis: Anatomy & Exercises,* by Blandine Calais-Germain (Seattle: Eastland Press, 2003).

Incontinence

Incontinence is the inability to stop the flow of urine when we want to. It can take several forms:

- Stress incontinence usually happens when too much pressure has been put on the perineum. It is most common in women over the age of forty, especially when the perineum has been taxed by pregnancy and childbirth.
- Urge incontinence—a frequent, urgent need to urinate, often accompanied by leakage of urine—is caused by spasms of the bladder muscles. It is most common in the elderly. It's also possible to suffer from fecal incontinence, in other words, to lose control of the bowels.

Putting intense pressure on the perineum while doing abdominal exercises can contribute to incontinence. This is why it's important to:

- Determine the intensity and amount of exercise based on the state of the perineum. If the perineum is weak, avoid exercises that are intense and, above all, exercises that send pressure downward toward the perineum.
- Always work the abdominals in coordination with the perineum.

Other Key Words

Muscle Soreness

After repeated intense exercise, a muscle or muscle group will sometimes feel sore. Generally, soreness appears the day after exercising. There are several reasons for this, but most often muscle soreness is caused by microscopic tearing of the muscle fibers—a necessary step in the strengthening of muscles.

Cramps

A cramp is a sudden, involuntary contraction or spasm of a muscle. It's usually painful, and it generally occurs while we're using the muscle. Often cramps are due to poor circulation within the muscle, which itself has many causes, including poor warm-up of muscle or the type of contraction. Cramps most often happen when doing isometric exercise.

Vascularization

The word *vascularization* denotes the network of vessels in an area of the body as well as the flow in those vessels: the circulation of blood in the arteries and veins, the circulation of lymphatic fluid in the lymphatic vessels, and so on.

Regarding vascularization in the abdominals, it's important that abdominal exercises encourage circulation to the core of the muscles so that they are properly nourished to avoid pain and cramping. We do this by:

- Alternating the direction of movement to recruit the muscle layers one after the other
- Varying the length of the muscle in the course of exercising

Fascia

Fascia is the fibrous connective tissue that we find throughout the body. Most often fascia

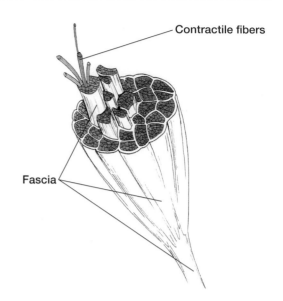

Contractile fibers

Fascia

surrounds soft structures like the viscera, as well as the muscles.

Fascia is neither elastic nor contractile. However, the fascia coming from a muscle can extend the effect of the muscle's contraction, even though it makes up the noncontractile part of the muscle. This is the case with the broad abdominal muscles, in which the contractile (red) fibers extend their reach to the front of the body by way of the white sheets of fascia. The fasciae from broad muscles that have a wide area of attachment at the front of the abdomen are sometimes called the aponeuroses.

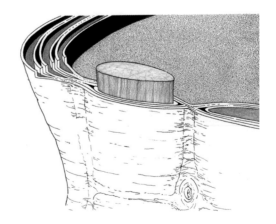

How the Abdominals Pull on the Linea Alba

Each of the broad muscles pulls its aponeurosis outward, back toward itself. The aponeurosis, not being contractile itself, can't counter this pull. It is neither extendable nor elastic, only deformable: it tightens under the effect of the contractile (red) fibers.

When the broad muscles on both sides of the abdomen contract at the same time, they pull the right aponeurosis to the right and the left aponeurosis to the left. The linea alba then finds itself being pulled apart.

The contraction of the transversus abdominis pulls on the aponeurosis that runs perpendicularly along the entire length of the linea alba. It tends to pull the linea alba apart, a little like a zipper splitting it in half.

The contraction of the obliques separates the linea alba obliquely.

So, the contraction of the three broad muscles exerts a strong pull that can separate the linea alba—a pull that is intensified when they are all working at the same time. This is the case when we try to pull the belly in on a forced exhalation. During this action the transversus abdominis, which is the strongest separator, is dominant.

The fibers of the rectus abdominis run parallel to the linea alba. Their contraction has no separating effect on the linea alba.

The contraction of the three broad muscles separates the linea alba. The rectus abdominis is the only abdominal muscle that does not separate the linea alba.

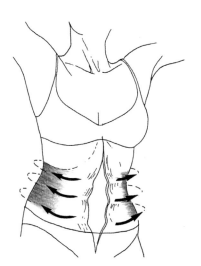

The transversus abdominis muscles separate the linea alba along its entire length.

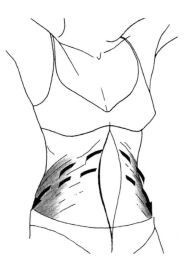

The internal obliques separate the linea alba principally in the upper region.

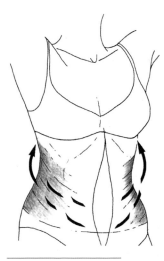

The external obliques separate the linea alba principally in the lower region.

PART TWO

Abdominal Strength versus a Flat Belly

✦ *Evaluating the Flat Belly*

✦ *Flat Belly and Protruding Belly*

✦ *A "User's Guide" to a Flat Belly*

✦ *Customized Strengthening Programs*

EVALUATING
THE FLAT BELLY

+ **False Evidence**

+ **Certain Abdominal Exercises Push the Belly Out**

+ **We Can Pull In the Belly without Contracting the Abdominals**

+ **Certain Abdominal Exercises Narrow the Waist
  but Don't Flatten the Belly**

+ **It's Not Good to Always Keep the Belly Flat**

+ **Pulling In the Belly: Consequences for the Perineum
  and the Prostate**

False Evidence

When we think of abdominal exercises, we think of a flat belly. The main reason that we work the abdominals is to improve our figure—to get or keep a flat belly. Out of 200 women who attended workshops on abdominal exercise, 197 responded that the main reason they wanted to practice abdominal exercises was to get, or to keep, their belly flat.

Yet abdominal exercises don't always make the belly flat!

• Certain exercises make the belly protrude (pages 41–42).

• We can pull in the belly very well without contracting the abdominals (page 42).

• Certain exercises can narrow the waist but do not flatten the belly (pages 42–43).

• It's not good to keep the belly flat all the time (page 43).

• Having a flat belly is not always a matter of the abdominals (pages 45–48).

• To get a flat belly, the abdominals have to be worked in a specific way (pages 49–54).

Certain Abdominal Exercises Push the Belly Out

Any movement that flexes the trunk pushes the bulk of the abdominal mass forward.

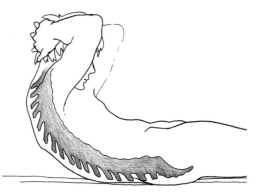

Flexing the trunk also closes the rib cage, so that the viscera located in the lower part of the rib cage are pushed forward.

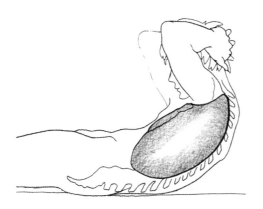

While doing an intense abdominal exercise, we tend to close the glottis to make the rib cage more compact and thus easier to move. Closing the glottis has the downside of sending the pressure downward toward the belly, so that the abdomen pooches.

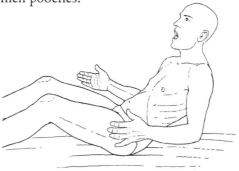

Sometimes we go even further: we close the glottis, and then we give an additional downward push (the action of the diaphragm).

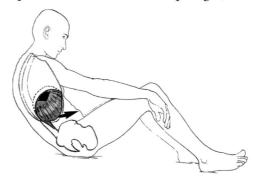

Important Note

Contraction of the abdominals can prevent the belly from being pushed out. However:

- First, a place has to be found for the displaced contents of the abdomen.
- Second, upon contraction of the abdominals, the upper belly can't be pushed down toward the pelvis.

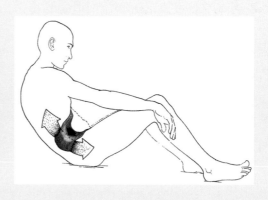

When doing abdominal exercises we are often asked to pull in our belly on a forceful exhalation. This recruits specifically the transversus abdominis. If we aren't told exactly where to pull in the belly, and in what direction, we tend to try to narrow the waist and just above the waist, forming an hourglass shape. This pushes the viscera toward the top and, even more, the bottom of the hourglass, pushing out the belly.

Important Note

Crunches (see pages 60–71) often combine all of these movements that push out the belly: the flexion of the trunk, closing of the rib cage, glottal stop, downward push of the diaphragm, and pulling in of the belly upon a forceful exhalation.

We Can Pull In the Belly without Contracting the Abdominals

To pull in the belly without contracting the abdominals, we need to open the rib cage. When we open the ribs like this, the rib cage takes on the form and the action of a suction cup: it pulls the viscera up with it, and the belly lifts and pulls in. This resembles the action of pulling in the belly, but it can be done with or without contracting the abdominals.

We can practice this movement by lifting our arms or uncurling our spine. It can be linked to an inhalation, but it doesn't need to be.

This effect is even more marked when we are lying down.

Certain Abdominal Exercises Narrow the Waist but Don't Flatten the Belly

The isolated contraction of the transversus abdominis reduces the diameter of the abdomen. This action is most noticeable at the waist, between the ribs and the pelvis, where the transversus muscle fibers are the longest and the most numerous.

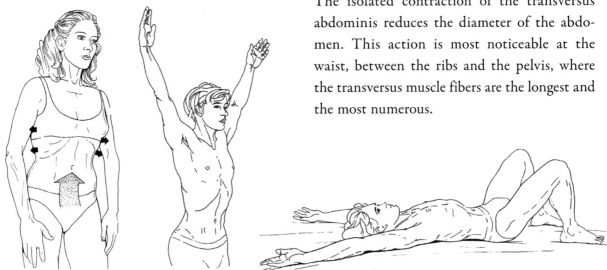

Opening the rib cage lifts the belly and pulls it in, with or without contraction of the abdominals.

When the transversus abdominis contracts, the waist takes on an hourglass form. The viscera in the contracted area are displaced upward to some degree, but mostly downward, away from the squeezed area. They can form a little pooch just below the contracted area. This effect is most apparent in a vertical position.

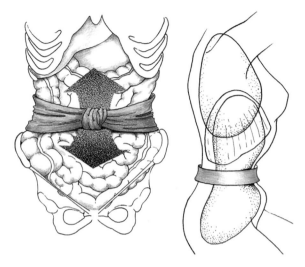

This movement is particularly noticeable when a person wears a belt at the waist that is too tight; in this situation we tend to pull in the transversus abdominis in a "beltlike" manner, which can leave a groove in the skin of the waist. Under the groove, the belly often pooches.

It's Not Good to Always Keep the Belly Flat

The abdominal muscles make up a part of the abdominal cavity, the container that surrounds the viscera of the abdomen. These organs perform varied functions, from digestion to circulation to elimination. Each of them alternately fill and empty at a rhythm that depends on their function, courtesy of a type of movement specific to the viscera: motility. For example, the intestines move the products of digestion thanks to alternating contractions of the intestinal walls.

For good digestion, it's important to:

- Exercise, which facilitates transit through the intestines. The simple act of changing position is a form of exercise that will move the intestines, and of course abdominal exercises are good for this as well, as long as they are varied.
- Relax the abdominals throughout the day. It's even helpful to massage the viscera with the abdominals relaxed. This is particularly beneficial after a meal—although this might best be done on your day off or when you're on vacation, as it might not be appropriate during the workday!

Keeping the abdominals constantly contracted can impede the motility and function of the viscera.

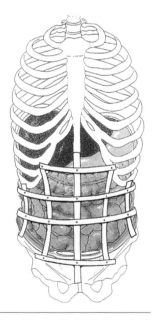

Keeping the belly flat at all times is too restrictive for the viscera.

Pulling In the Belly:
Consequences for the Perineum and the Prostate

Pulling In the Belly Increases Pressure on the Perineum

To totally flatten our belly, we contract all of the abdominals. Since the contents of the abdomen are thereby restrained from being at the front of the abdomen, they move up or down. This has the unfortunate side effect of putting additional pressure on the perineum.

When we practice diaphragmatic breathing and try to pull in our belly at the same time, the push of the diaphragm is not compensated for by expansion of the belly. Instead, the belly moves to the sides and down toward the perineum. This also increases the pressure on the viscera of the small pelvis.

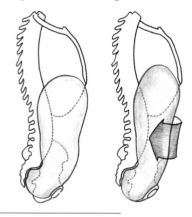

Flattening the belly displaces the viscera and puts pressure on the perineum.

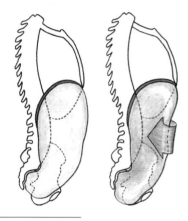

Pulling in the belly while practicing diaphragmatic breathing increases the pressure on the perineum.

Keeping the Belly Pulled In Compresses the Prostate

Unlike the female pelvic floor, the male pelvic floor doesn't have an opening in it. And since the pelvic floor is closed, it is not able to compensate for increased pressure by creating a prolapse, like it might in a woman.

The male pelvic floor is also smaller in size than a female's, and therefore less capable of changing shape. When abdominal exercise creates downward pressure, the male pelvic floor responds by sending pressure in the other direction, from low to high. The prostate finds itself squeezed in between.

Pulling in the belly can increase pressure on the perineum.

If you are male, when working the abdominals, it's best to focus on drawing pressure away from the perineum by keeping the ribs open or by coordinating the abdominal contraction from the bottom up.

If you're female, look to tone the pelvic floor in addition to lessening the pressure on it.

FLAT BELLY AND PROTRUDING BELLY

✦ It's Not Just a Matter of Muscles

✦ Fat and the Flat Belly

✦ A Thorax That Does or Does Not Weigh on the Abdomen

✦ A Spine That Does or Does Not Push the Abdomen Downward

It's Not Just a Matter of Muscles

The Nine Factors behind a Flat Belly

1. Little or no fat between the skin and the abdominals (subcutaneous fat)
2. Little or no fat between the viscera (intra-abdominal fat)
3. A certain way of inhaling with the ribs
4. A certain way of exhaling with the abdomen
5. A thorax that doesn't weigh on the abdomen
6. A spine that doesn't push the abdomen downward
7. Abdominal strength
8. Coordination of the abdominals
9. Good elimination

The Nine Factors behind a Protruding Belly

1. Fat between the skin and the abdominals
2. Fat between the viscera (intra-abdominal fat)
3. A certain way of inhaling with the diaphragm
4. A certain way of exhaling with the ribs
5. A thorax that weighs on the abdomen
6. A spine that pushes the abdominals downward
7. Abdominal weakness
8. Lack of coordination of the abdominals
9. Intestinal flatulence

Fat and a Flat Belly

Fat accumulates easily around the midsection. To lose it, we can:

• Experiment with food intake (go on a diet or, better yet, eat a balanced diet)

• Exercise, which contributes to burning fat (this includes abdominal exercise)

• Resort to surgery (where fat is removed by liposuction)

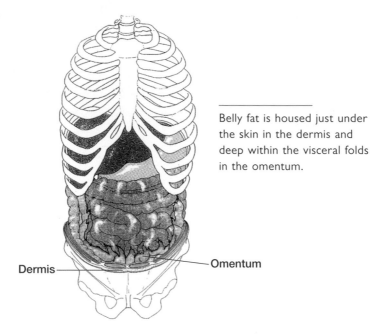

Belly fat is housed just under the skin in the dermis and deep within the visceral folds in the omentum.

Dermis — — Omentum

Specific actions relate to where the fat accumulates, and how we can get rid of it.

Fat between the Viscera

The abdominal viscera are contained in a membrane called the peritoneum. This membrane folds back on itself in several areas deep in the coils of the intestines. A large fold in front of the intestines is called the omentum or epiploon. Fat is often housed in the omentum and other deep folds of the peritoneum.

To lose this fat, we can:

- Mobilize the viscera with specific exercises
- Massage the viscera

Fat under the Skin

The skin is made up of two principal layers:

- The epidermis, which we can see and touch. It's the most superficial layer.

- The dermis, which is deeper and thicker. It's the most vital layer. The deepest layer of the dermis is the hypodermis, which contains the cells that can most readily store fat: the adipocytes.

When we gain weight, the fat accumulates in the hypodermis in specific areas of the body, and in particular in the anterior walls of the belly.

To get rid of this fat, we can:

- Massage the areas of the skin where the fat accumulates to mobilize it.
- Stretch specific muscles, such as the external obliques and the rectus abdominis, that lie just under the skin.

When it comes to fighting fat, exercising the abdominal muscles has only an indirect effect; all physical exercise helps burn fat.

A Thorax That Does or Does Not Weigh on the Abdomen

Closing the rib cage causes two things to happen:

- The diameter of the thorax decreases because the sternum is brought closer to the spine, creating less space for everything that is contained in the rib cage. The contents are forced downward toward the abdomen.
- The capacity of the upper rib cage decreases, which redirects the viscera of the thorax toward the abdomen. The organs of the thorax have to move downward, and they tend to move toward the abdomen. The belly then sticks out, putting pressure on the abdominal wall.

> For the belly to be flat,
> the rib cage must be open.

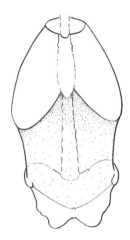 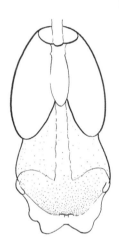 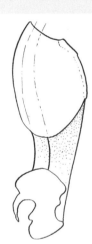 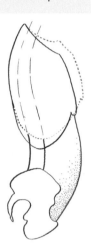

A Spine That Does or Does Not Push the Abdomen Downward

When we flex the spine forward, the viscera are pushed together and moved forward, pushing the belly out.

If spinal flexion takes the pelvis closer to the throat (flexion from the tail), the viscera are pushed up toward the thorax. If we eat before making this motion, it can even provoke reflux.

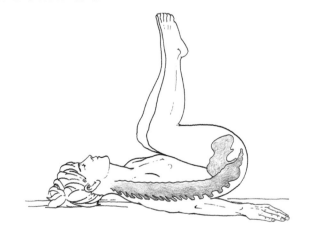

If spinal flexion takes the throat toward the pelvis (flexion from the head), the viscera are sent down toward the pelvis. When we are standing, this displacement of the viscera will be more intense thanks to the pull of gravity.

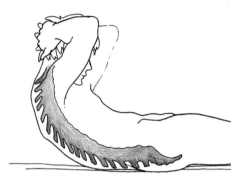

The spine and rib cage often move together. Flexion of the spine is often associated with the ribs dropping. (The two movements tend to be spontaneously synchronized.) This synchronization contributes to pushing the viscera toward the pelvis.

Standing Posture and a Flat Belly

A standing position with the back rounded (kyphosis) tends to cause the belly to pooch out.

Simply realigning the spine, with no thought of contracting the abdominals, helps prevent a pooching belly.

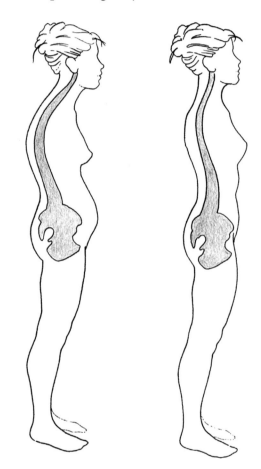

A "USER'S GUIDE"
TO A FLAT BELLY

* Alternately Stretch and Contract the Abdominals
* Alternately Contract the Broad Muscles
* Alternately Contract the Broad Muscles and Rectus Abdominis
* Coordinate Abdominal Contractions
* Coordinate Abdominal Work with the Breath

Alternately Stretch and Contract the Abdominals

When we alternate the stretching and contraction of a muscle, the contractile fibers of the muscle change in shape and volume, and this movement of the tissue promotes blood circulation to the core of the muscle.

The recommended exercises in part 4 of this book often alternate stretching and con-traction of the abdominal muscles. In a contraction, the contractile (red) fibers of the muscle shorten and thicken, while the white noncontractile fibers (tendon or aponeurosis) are put under tension. In a stretch, both the contractile and noncontractile tissues are put under tension.

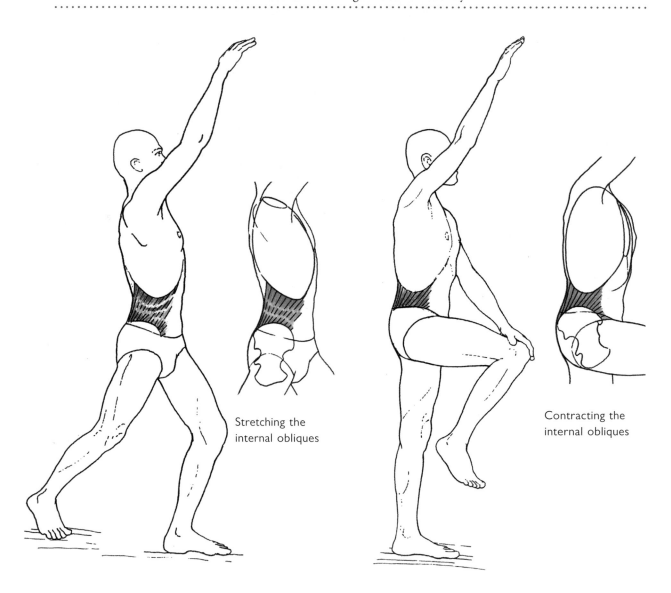

Stretching the
internal obliques

Contracting the
internal obliques

Alternately Contract the Broad Muscles

The broad muscles, in a three-layer latticework, adhere a bit to each other by way of their fascia "envelopes."

When one of the obliques contracts preferentially in an exercise, it draws the other two layers of muscle along with it, in the direction of its contraction. This changes the form of the other two muscles, whose fibers don't run in the same direction. They are "massaged" a little,

like a towel being twisted. If on the next contraction we focus on another oblique, the same phenomenon occurs, and all three layers move in another direction.

When we alternate the contractions of the broad muscles (obliques and transversus abdominis) in this way, the sliding/massaging that it causes stimulates circulation, which nourishes the tissues.

The suggested exercises at the end of this book often alternate the contraction of the broad muscles.

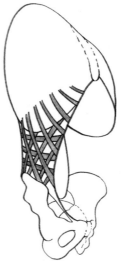

The broad muscles form a three-layer latticework.

Alternately Contract the Broad Muscles and Rectus Abdominis

The broad muscles pull the anterior aponeurosis to the sides, putting it under lateral tension.

The rectus abdominis, when contracted, shortens from top to bottom along the length of the belly. It pulls the anterior aponeurosis upward and downward, in the same direction as its fibers.

Alternating the direction of traction in this way promotes mobility and good elimination in the tissues that are being stretched.

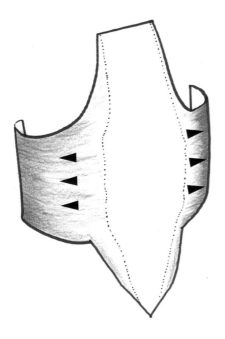

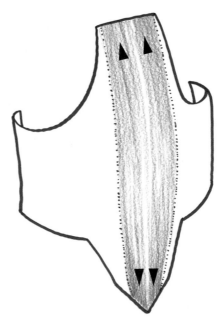

Coordinate Abdominal Contractions

Each of the abdominals can contract in its entirety or only in part because these muscles are innervated by different groups of nerves.

We can contract the abdominals in stages at precise levels. For example, we can pull in just the upper belly, the mid-belly, or the lower belly. It's good to try this just to note that it is indeed possible and even easy.

We can also combine contractions to pull the belly in successive stages in one direction. This will push the abdominal mass in a given direction, a little like pushing toothpaste in a tube from one end to the other. Certain contraction combinations are more interesting than others.

If we start pulling the belly in at the top and work downward, we push the belly toward the pelvis. But if we start the contraction from the bottom and work upward, this pushes the belly up. If we're looking for a flat belly, the best way to work is with this type of "ascending contraction."

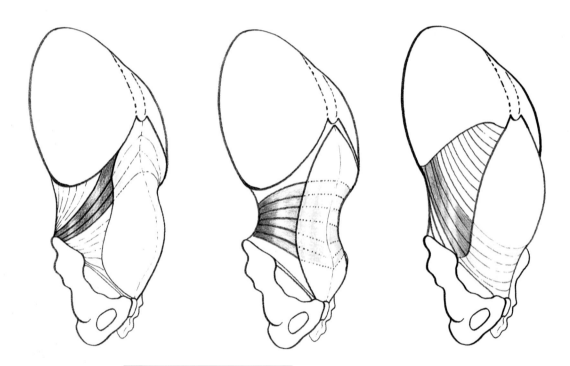

We can pull in just the upper belly, the mid-belly, or the lower belly.

Coordinate Abdominal Work with the Breath

A detailed study of the various ways in which we can coordinate abdominal work and the breath are not within the scope of this work. Basically, what we will look at here are two principal types of inhalation and exhalation.

An inhalation may be diaphragmatic, which will cause the belly to expand, or costal (with the ribs), which tends to pull the belly in.

When we are doing abdominal work on an inhalation, it's best to choose costal breathing. This is what we propose in the exercises at the end of this book.

An exhalation can be costal, which lowers the ribs and can push out the belly, or abdominal, which brings the abdomen up toward the thorax and can cause the belly to pull in.

When we practice abdominal exercises on an exhalation, it's best to choose an abdominal exhalation. This is what we propose in the exercises in this book.

However, abdominal work often naturally imposes its own breathing pattern: it generally closes the ribs, and so we tend to associate abs work with a costal exhalation. The reverse is not spontaneous and therefore takes a bit of practice.

> If you contract the abdominals on an exhalation, it's important that the exhalation be accompanied by a lifting of the abdomen and not by a closing of the ribs.

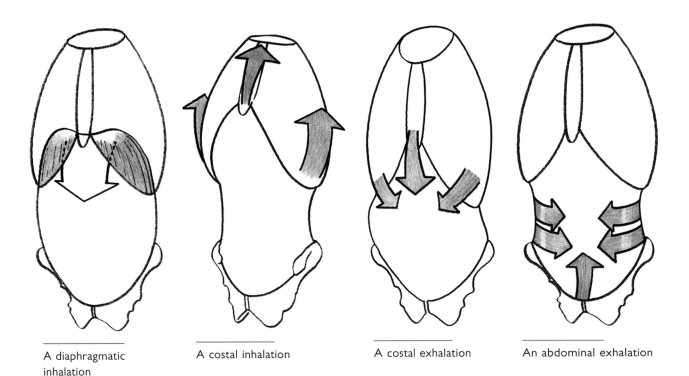

A diaphragmatic inhalation

A costal inhalation

A costal exhalation

An abdominal exhalation

Important Note

In general, when we do an abdominal exercise, "visceral synchronization" most often follows the dominant pattern of "skeletal synchronization." For example, when doing a crunch, we roll the spine from top to bottom, and we tend to contract the abdominals in the same direction, from high to low. This is not desirable for the perineum or for the walls of the abdomen. It would be better, when the movement moves from top to bottom, to coordinate this with an "ascending contraction." However, this is difficult because the movements run counter to each other.

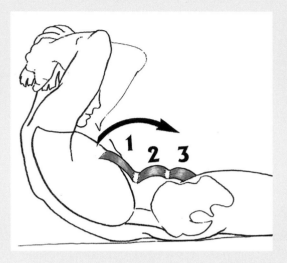

A crunch tends to contract the abdominals from top to bottom.

CUSTOMIZED STRENGTHENING PROGRAMS

✦ Individual Strength and Customized Training

Individual Strength and Customized Training

Abdominal strength alone doesn't determine how flat the belly will be. And giving priority to muscle development for that purpose has inherent risks. However, if the abdominals are weak, it does make sense to strengthen them.

As with all muscles, the abdominals will strengthen as a result of adopting a system of muscle toning or building. The fundamental principle of these systems is always the same: you have to contract the muscles against a resistance that is greater than what they are used to.

Important Note

Muscle toning or building has nothing to do with stretching exercises and methods to increase flexibility. It also does not relate to relaxation techniques and movement coordination. This is strictly related to building muscle strength.

Strength training is necessarily customized based on the individual, because greater resistance than the muscles are accustomed to is not the same for everybody. Resistance needs to be greater for someone who exercises regularly (a professional dancer or athlete) than for someone who exercises moderately (someone who spends a couple of hours a week at the gym). The resistance is going to be even less for someone who never exercises or is very weak (an infirm or older individual). We should note that even among people in the same group, the level of resistance will vary greatly. It will even vary from one day to the next for each person. Each of us needs to be mindful of what constitutes the appropriate amount of force for our body. It's very important to monitor the amount of force and resistance we use when participating in a group class designed to strengthen the abs. The same awareness applies when we are working out on machines or working along with a book or video. The necessary level of resistance is not the same for everyone!

How do you determine the appropriate level of resistance for you? You can work with a professional who can tell you how many exercise repetitions to do and how to adjust the resistance on a particular machine. If your breathing accelerates and your heart starts beating faster while you are exercising, you are probably stressing your muscles more than you are accustomed to. Don't force yourself. Look to make steady and gradual progress from session to session. If you feel muscle pain between sessions, perhaps the sessions have been too intense. Pay more attention to the time between muscle contraction and decontraction and make sure that you're breathing properly.

PART THREE

The Five Most Common Abdominal Exercises

- ✦ *Working the Abdominals*
- ✦ *Crunches*
- ✦ *Leg Lifts*
- ✦ *Push-ups*
- ✦ *Supine Trunk Rotation*
- ✦ *Pulling In the Belly on a Forceful Exhalation*

WORKING THE ABDOMINALS

✦ The Basic Anatomical "Recipe"

✦ How Do We Create or Increase Resistance?

✦ What Are the Inherent Risks in Abdominal Exercises?

The Basic Anatomical "Recipe"

The basic principles of working the abdominals are always the same.

We must fix or mobilize the areas of the trunk to which the abdominals are attached:

- The pelvis

- The ribs
- The lumbar spine or lumbothoracic spine.

We must create or augment resistance to an abdominal movement, making it more difficult (see pages 55–56).

How Do We Create or Increase Resistance?

Resistance is created or increased for the abdominals during an exercise by the following:

- The weight of the head pulling on the rib cage (see the text on rolling up from the head toward the thorax on page 61)
- The weight of the head and the thorax pulling on the rib cage (see the text on rolling the thorax toward the abdomen on page 61)
- The weight of the head, the thorax, and the abdomen pulling on the pelvis (see the text on rolling the upper body toward the pelvis on page 61)
- The weight of the arms, which makes the exercise more intense
- The weight of the legs, which pull on the pelvis (see leg lift text on pages 73 and 85)
- Resistance from a partner or piece of equipment
- Resistance from pressure on or anchoring of a part of the body

What Are the Inherent Risks in Abdominal Exercises?

Risks for the following anatomical areas are detailed on the pages listed:

- The perineum—see pages 65, 81–82, and 90

- The walls of the abdomen, with the risk of hernias—see pages 62–63
- The lumbar and thoracic intervertebral disks—see pages 66–67, 69, 78, 82, and 86
- The cervical intervertebral disks—see pages 70–71

CRUNCHES

The Basic Crunch

1. Lie down on your back, with your knees bent and feet flat on the floor.
2. Roll up your head, then your neck, your shoulders, and your rib cage. Finally, come to a seated position, bringing your upper body toward your legs.

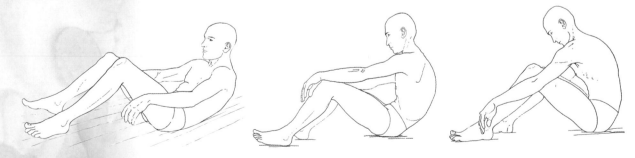

The exercise can be done by rolling straight up or by coming up a bit to the right or the left.

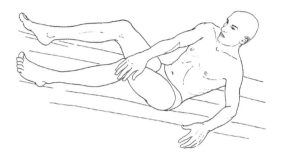

How Crunches Work the Abs

In a crunch, the abdominal muscles work in four stages, in different ways:

Stage 1 • Head Lifted
Only the head is lifted. This movement is initiated by the neck flexors, which insert on the rib cage. The abdominals contract to keep the rib cage aligned with the pelvis. This action is called fixation, or a static or isometric contraction.

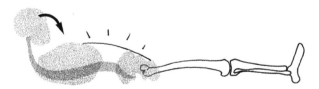

Stage 2 • Head and Shoulders Lifted
The head and shoulders are lifted (with or without the arms). The abdominals still contract to keep the rib cage over the pelvis, but now with more intensity. This is still a fixation action; the abdominals don't move the skeleton.

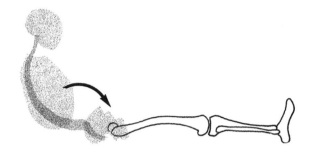

Stage 3 • Shoulder Blades and Ribs Lifted
As the shoulder blades and the back ribs lift off the floor, the abdominals contract to roll the rib cage toward the abdominals. This contraction to initiate a movement is called mobilization, or a concentric contraction.

Stage 4 • Whole Torso Lifted
If the crunch continues and brings the whole torso and head up toward the thighs, it does so by a contraction of the hip flexors. At this stage, the abdominals work again to keep the torso between the rib cage and the pelvis. They don't pull the torso to the pelvis.

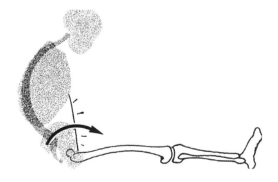

During the roll-down phase of the crunch, the abdominal muscles work as much as they do in the roll-up. They work for different reasons at each stage, but most often in a static mode. This doesn't encourage good blood circulation. You might say that the muscles are "suffocated" during the exercise. So it would not be surprising to be sore the next day (see pages 35–36).

Crunches Can Vary in Intensity

The rib cage and the head are very heavy. Because of this weight, a crunch is an extreme exercise. It gets more and more intense:

- The higher we raise our trunk
- The closer we bring our body to our feet
- When we don't help ourselves up by essentially pitching ourselves forward with our arms

Crunches Can Endanger the Abdominal Walls

1 • Pushing the Viscera Down

In a crunch, we roll the upper part of the trunk over the lower part, bringing the rib cage toward the pelvis. This pushes the viscera down in the same direction.

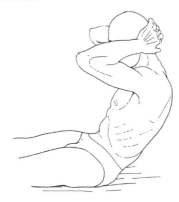

2 • Flattening the Rib Cage

The abdominals tend to close the ribs during a crunch, flattening the rib cage. This drives the contents of the thorax downward.

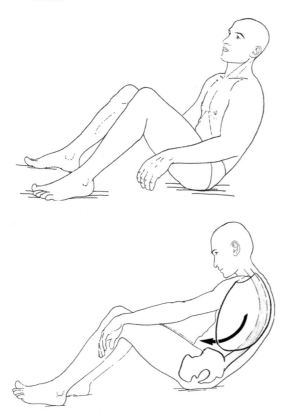

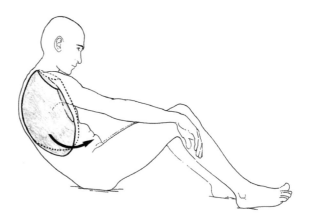

3 • *Closing the Glottis*

To minimize the closing of the rib cage during a crunch, we sometimes close the glottis, blocking our breath. This does keep the rib cage more open, but it has the downside of putting pressure on the abdominal wall, which will then push outward.

4 • *Pushing with the Glottis Closed*

With the glottis closed, we will sometimes "push" against it during a crunch. This contraction of the diaphragm causes the belly to bulge even more. Though this pushing is a natural response to closing the glottis, it doesn't actually facilitate the movement of the crunch.

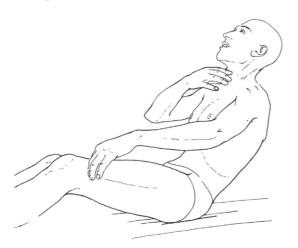 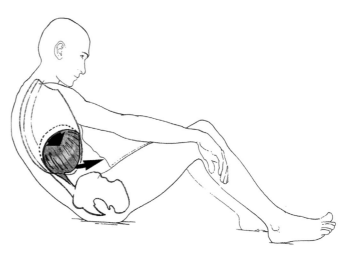

A crunch is intense because the upper body is heavy to lift and roll up. The four issues mentioned above often come into play when we try to perform a crunch. If so, the abdominal wall can be compromised, especially if it is fragile (with disk herniations and linea alba distension issues). For a woman who has just given birth, this kind of abdominal exercise is contraindicated.

Making Crunches Safer for the Abdominal Walls

Protecting the Abdominal Walls

- Avoid closing the glottis and "pushing." Work with the glottis open. The best way to keep the glottis open is to keep breathing.
- Avoid closing the ribs. Open the ribs before starting the crunch. Keep the ribs wide for the entire roll-up and for the roll-down as well.

Aim to hollow the upper belly for the entire exercise, whether you are inhaling or exhaling (see pages 65–66).

Protecting the Linea Alba

- Avoid engaging the transversus abdominis, since it pulls strongly on the linea alba (see page 37).
- Avoid exhaling during the exercise, particularly an intense exhalation (which engages the transversus abdominis for the most part; see page 88). An intense exhalation, sometimes called a forced exhalation, is when we push out more air than in a normal exhalation and we go into what's called the expiratory reserve volume (ERV). For more details, see *Anatomy of Breathing,* by Blandine Calais-Germain (Seattle: Eastland Press, 2006).

Important Note

You might want to exhale during the exercise (since you flatten the ribs). So you have to start exhaling before rolling up, and start rolling up on the inhale.

Perform a crunch on an inhalation into the ribs. Exhale deeply before starting the movement, and inhale, opening the ribs, during the movement.

Crunches Can Endanger the Perineum

All the points listed on pages 62–63 can be applied to the pelvic floor.

1 • Pushing the Viscera Down

During a crunch, we roll the upper part of the torso over the lower part. The rib cage comes over the pelvis, which pushes the viscera down.

2 • Flattening the Rib Cage

The abs responsible for rolling up the body tend to close the ribs, flattening the rib cage. This contributes to driving the contents of the thorax toward the perineum.

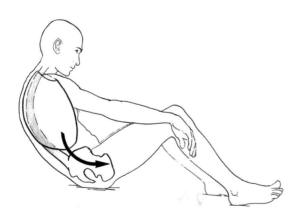

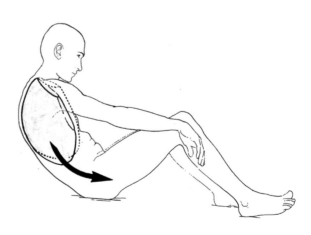

3 • *Closing the Glottis*

To minimize the closing of the rib cage, we tend to close the glottis, which blocks our breath. This does keep the rib cage from closing, but at the same time it pushes the viscera down toward the perineum.

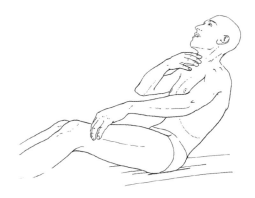

4 • *Pushing with the Glottis Closed*

Sometimes we even "push" with the glottis closed during a crunch. This contraction of the diaphragm puts even more pressure downward. Though this pushing is a natural response to closing the glottis, it doesn't actually facilitate the movement of the crunch.

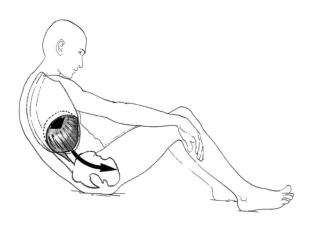

5 • *Pulling in the Belly*

We can add a fifth point: If we try to pull the belly in by contracting the abs, the visceral mass can't stay in the front part of the abdomen. It has to spread elsewhere, moving toward the top but also toward the "small pelvis." This makes the pressure on the perineum even stronger.

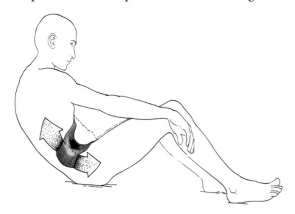

Crunches with the belly pulled in may increase the pressure on the perineum. They can cause prolapse or compress the prostate. Avoid crunches if you have a weak perineum.

Making Crunches Safer for the Perineum

It's not easy to protect the perineum while doing crunches because many different actions must be coordinated. If you are not well trained, it's better to choose other exercises. If you are used to doing crunches and still want to practice them, here are some useful tips.

Avoid Closing the Ribs

Before doing crunches, get the ribs moving (see pages 102–4).

- Try to open the ribs as wide as possible, especially in the back part of the rib cage.
- Open the ribs and inhale as you start rolling up.
- Keep the ribs wide while rolling up.

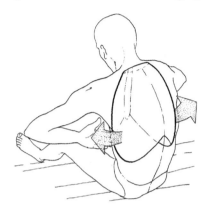

Hollow the Top Part of the Belly during the Exercise

This "hollowing" doesn't come from any action of the abdominals but from the ribs widening. Don't try to pull the rest of the belly in.

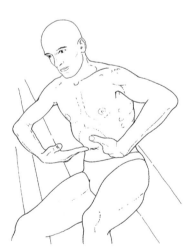

To protect the perineum, it's much better to do crunches on an inhalation rather than on a exhalation, and more specifically on a costal inhalation avoiding closing the glottis during the whole exercise. Don't try to pull the belly in, except the top part of the belly, which is pulled in by opening the ribs.

Crunches Can Endanger the Lumbar Disks in Flexion

In the fourth stage of the crunch, we lift the head, trunk, and pelvis in flexion to the thighs. This movement demands a strong contraction of the hip flexors. But the hip flexors tend for the most part to flex the thigh to the trunk.

Anchoring the Feet

At this stage of the crunch, certain people can't complete the movement without their feet being held (by another person or by anchoring their feet under something). If they don't have pressure on their feet, their legs lift, and their trunk falls backward.

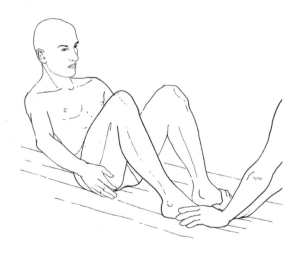

If they can complete the movement with their feet being held, the strength of their abdominals is not the cause of their inability to complete the movement without their feet being held. Neither is the mobility of their spine a major factor (this can be tested; see the following page).

Body Proportions

The major cause is one of body proportions: the weight of the legs balances the weight of the trunk. This is true of people who have a long trunk and short legs. They are at a great disadvantage in this exercise.

For those who have a short trunk and long legs, the opposite is the case.

People who are at a disadvantage when doing crunches—those with a long trunk and short legs—tend to throw themselves forward using their arms. They then overflex the lower part of the trunk in an attempt to lift the pelvis. This puts pressure on the lumbar disks, especially if they are asked to hold themselves at this critical point.

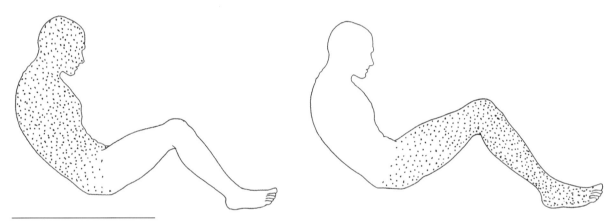

People with a long trunk and short legs are at a disadvantage when doing crunches. The opposite is true for those with a short trunk and long legs.

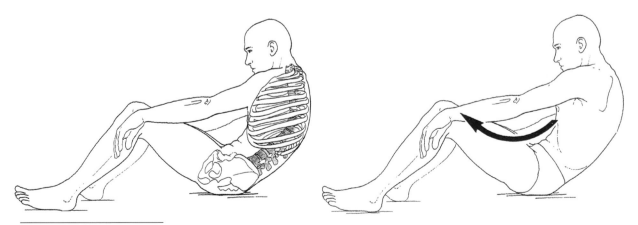

Those who are at a disadvantage tend to throw themselves forward with their arms and overflex the lower trunk.

Protecting the Lumbar Disks in Flexion

If you can't easily roll your trunk toward your legs, especially at the fourth stage of the crunch, without your feet being held, you should test the flexion of your lumbar spine:

- Lie on your side in a fetal position.
- Pull your knees in toward your belly and your thorax toward your knees.

If you cannot make this movement easily, it's best to use safe flexion exercises to loosen up the spine.

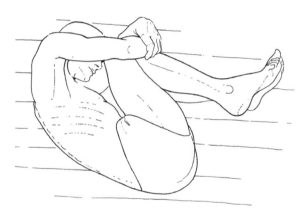

Next, test the crunch with your feet being held, either:

- By someone else
- By anchoring your feet under a heavy bar, piece of furniture, et cetera

This way you can verify whether abdominal strength is the problem.

If the tests show that the spine is mobile and the abdominals are strong enough, you most likely have a problem of body proportions, and you must avoid putting pressure on your lumbar disks by overflexing the spine. How?

- Work just that part of the crunch with your feet held.
- Avoid coming straight up, and instead roll up slightly to one side of the trunk (alternating sides).

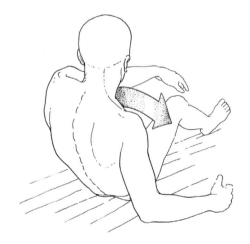

Important Note

To make the spine more supple in flexion, it's best to practice exercises that don't put too much pressure on the disks. See *Anatomy of Movement: Exercises,* by Blandine Calais-Germain and Andrée Lamotte (Seattle: Eastland Press, 2008).

Crunches Can Endanger the Lumbar Disks in Extension

In the fourth stage of the crunch, we lift the head, trunk, and pelvis in flexion to the thighs. This movement calls for a strong contraction of the hip flexors. Here we run the risk of the hip flexors pulling the pelvis into anteversion, arching the lumbar spine.

It's not the arching of the lumbar spine that puts the disks at risk, but the strong compression that is caused by the action of the hip flexors and the abdominals in this movement.

This compression can overstress the lumbar disks, especially if we repeat the exercise or hold the spine in this arched position (because this is the most difficult part of the exercise).

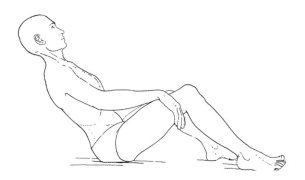

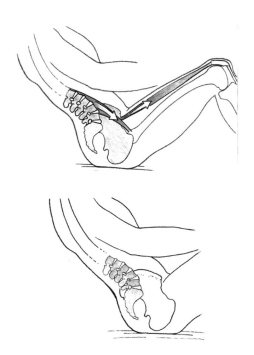

Important Note

The arching of the lower back (extension) can occur in the same movement as hyperflexion. The spine will "hesitate" between the two positions, putting even more pressure on the disks. This will overstress the lumbar disks, especially if we repeat the exercise or hold this precarious position.

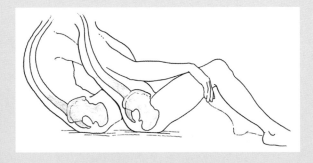

Protecting the Lumbar Disks in Extension

If you don't need to have your feet held down to complete a crunch (and body proportions are favorable; see page 67), it's best to avoid doing this, as fixing the feet turns the crunch into just an exercise for the hip flexors.

If you do need to have your feet held in order to do a crunch, you may tend to arch your back as you roll up. If this is the case, it's better not to come straight up, but to tilt a bit to the side. This means more work for the lateral abdominals (obliques) and prevents a lumbar arch.

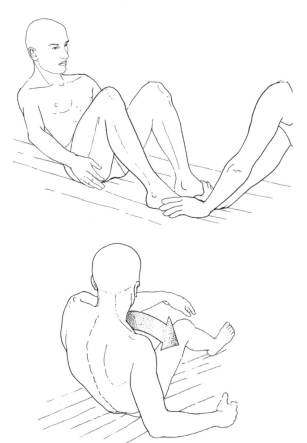

Crunches Can Endanger the Cervical Disks

We sometimes place our hands behind our head when doing a crunch. We do this for two very different reasons:

- We look to intensify the exercise by avoiding launching ourselves forward with our arms.
- We attempt to pull our head forward using the weight and muscular strength of our arms. This is most common, in light of the difficulty of the exercise. In this case, we tend to bring our elbows very far forward. More than anything, this causes a forceful flexion of the lower cervical spine.

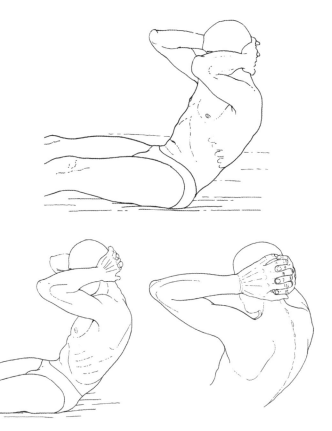

The hands pulling on the neck put the vertebrae of the lower cervical spine, which are very flexible, under a tremendous amount of pressure.

Protecting the Cervical Disks

Do not do crunches with your hands behind your head unless you have very strong abdominals and body proportions that favor the movement. If you do not have the right body proportions to accomplish the fourth stage of the crunch (see page 67), you'll need to have your feet held down, which will help you avoid pulling your neck into extreme flexion during a step that is too difficult for your body to accomplish.

If you want to do crunches with your hands behind your head, keep your elbows held out to the sides during this exercise, and verify that your head rests in your hands, instead of your hands resting or pulling on your head. If need be, you can hold your hands slightly away from your head.

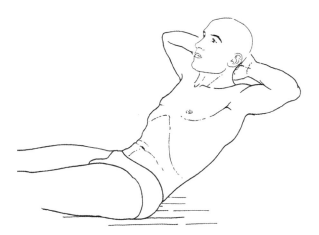

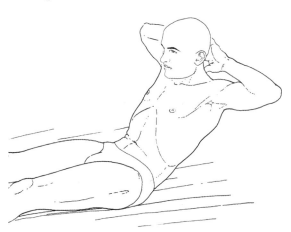

Important Note

Caution! You can pull your head forward (stressing the cervical disks) with your elbows held out to the sides just as you can with your elbows bent forward.

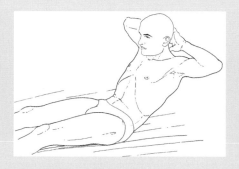

LEG LIFTS

✦ The Basic Leg Lift

✦ How Leg Lifts Work the Abdominals

✦ Leg Lifts Can Vary in Intensity

✦ The Pelvic Tipping Point: Retroversion versus Anteversion

✦ Leg Lifts Can Target Specific Abdominal Muscles

✦ Leg Lifts Can Endanger the Lumbar Spine

✦ Protecting the Lumbar Spine

The Basic Leg Lift

The Standard Lift

1. Lie down on your back.
2. Bring your legs up toward the ceiling.

Variations

- Keep your knees straight or bent.
- Lift your legs to a more vertical or less vertical position.
- Perform the exercise with one or both legs.
- Lift your legs to the front of your trunk or to one side or the other.

- Once you've lifted your legs, you can make a bicycling or scissoring movement, draw shapes, write your name, et cetera.

The many variations of the leg lift change:

- The intensity of the exercise
- The abdominals that are worked

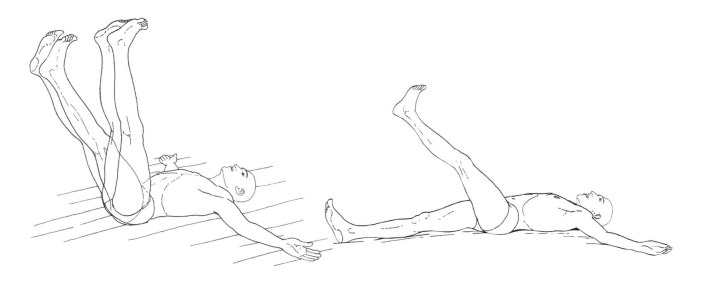

How Leg Lifts Work the Abdominals

The first thing that we need to understand about leg lifts is that it's not the abdominals that lift the legs, but the hip flexors (primarily the psoas, iliacus, sartorius, and tensor fascia latae muscles).

1 • The Hip Flexors Create Anteversion

The hip flexors don't just lift the legs; the fact that they are attached to the pelvis means that at the same moment they pull the pelvis into anteversion.

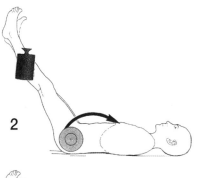

2 • The Abs Prevent Anteversion

It's here that the abdominals intervene to prevent the anteversion of the pelvis.

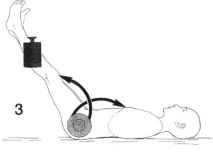

3 • The Abs Stabilize the Pelvis

The job of the abdominals is therefore to stabilize and fix the pelvis.

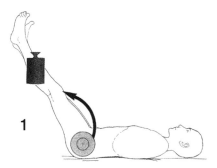

Important Note

The abdominal contraction that stabilizes the pelvis is a static or isometric contraction.

However, if we increase the amplitude of hip flexion, the pelvis tends to retrovert. This is why the action of the pelvis is sometimes opposite to the course of a movement (see pages 75–76).

Leg Lifts Can Vary in Intensity

Lifting one leg is much easier than lifting both legs. This difference is easy to feel. Trying to lift just one leg is a good way to see whether you can stabilize the pelvis while doing this exercise.

The exercise is also easier if the leg that is not lifted is pushed into the floor. This helps stabilize the pelvis. If you don't press the supporting leg into the floor, greater abdominal strength is required to lift the other leg.

A leg lift is much easier when the leg is bent rather than straight. If you think of the leg as a lever, the fulcrum is at the hip. Bending the leg essentially halves the length of the lever that the muscles must raise at the fulcrum. Because bending brings the weight of the leg closer to the body, less strength is required to lift it.

But there's another aspect at play here: Straight legs pull on hamstrings, found at the back of the thighs. The straighter the legs, and the closer they are pulled to the trunk, the more difficult the exercise becomes for the hamstrings, which work in the opposite direction. These muscles are progressively put under greater tension and brake the action of hip flexion. It's then necessary to increase the contraction of the hip flexors and also the contraction of the abdominals to fix the pelvis.

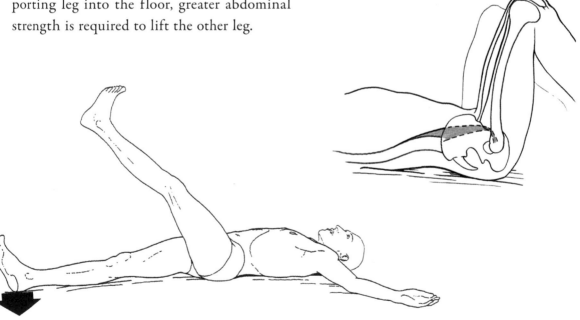

The angle of hip flexion changes the intensity of the exercise. The lower the leg drops—further from the vertical line of gravity—the more difficult the exercise becomes. We can easily feel that holding the legs just off the ground requires much more effort (for the hip flexors) than holding them in a vertical position. The pelvis is pulled more strongly into anteversion, and so the abdominals must work harder to stabilize it.

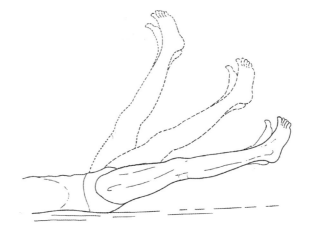

With leg lifts, we can start with the easiest variations and move to the more difficult ones.

The easiest variation is to lift just one leg, with the leg bent, to the point where the hip flexes at a ninety-degree angle (so that the leg is more or less vertical), while pushing the supporting leg into the floor.

The most difficult variation would be to lift both legs at the same time, with the legs straight and held very close to the floor.

The Pelvic Tipping Point: Retroversion versus Anteversion

1 • Retroversion
Lie on your back with your knees bent, bringing them as close as you can to your chest. Feel how your coccyx lifts from the floor and your pelvis goes into retroversion.

2 • Anteversion
Very slowly lower one leg toward the floor. On the side of the leg that is lowering, feel how that side of the pelvis changes position: from retroversion, it suddenly rocks into anteversion.

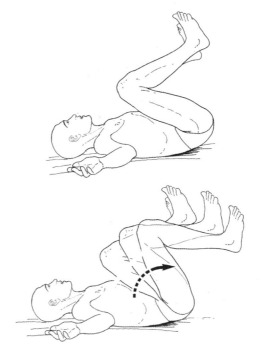

3 • The Tipping Point

Next, lower both bent legs slowly toward the floor. Feel the moment at which the whole pelvis moves from retroversion to anteversion. This is the "tipping point." It corresponds to a certain angle of hip flexion. Return several times to that precise point where the pelvis changes position.

Looking at the pelvis, we can say that any movement that occurs before the tipping point is retroversion, and any movement that occurs beyond the tipping point is anteversion.

Why does the pelvis go into retroversion when we bring our knees to our chest? The extreme hip flexion pulls the muscles and the ligaments at the back of the hips. When under tension, they pull the pelvis into retroversion.

Why does the pelvis go into anteversion when we bring our knees back toward the floor? When we extend our hips, the muscles at the front of the hips support the weight of the legs. The contraction of these muscles pulls the pelvis into anteversion.

Leg Lifts Can Target Specific Abdominal Muscles

If we raise the legs symmetrically, the pelvis moves into retroversion and the two sides of the pelvis are balanced. The rectus abdominis is the dominant player here as it retroverts the pelvis.

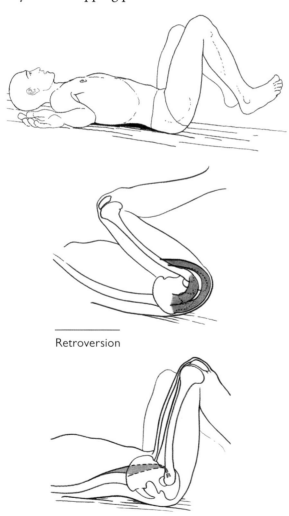

Retroversion

Anteversion

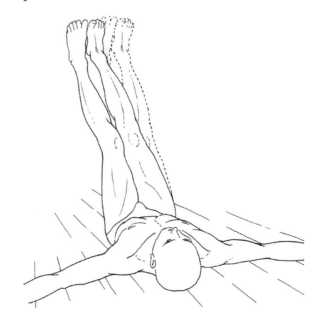

If the movement is asymmetrical, one side of the pelvis will move toward anteversion. For example:

- If we raise just one leg
- If we drop one or both legs a bit to one side
- If we scissor the legs, draw shapes in the air with our feet, et cetera

In all of these cases, the pelvis will turn to the side that is dominated by the movement of the legs. Therefore, to stabilize the pelvis, we need to suppress anteversion (the work of the rectus abdominis) and also inhibit rotation (the work of the obliques).

The work of the obliques can vary in intensity (see pages 72–75).

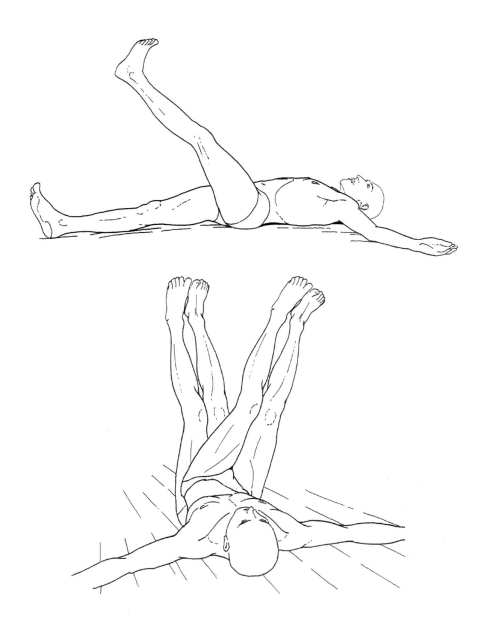

Leg Lifts Can Endanger the Lumbar Spine

1 • *Flexion*

When we bend our knees and bring them toward our chest (before the tipping point; see pages 75–76), the pelvis pulls the lumbar spine into flexion. This stretches the muscles and ligaments of the back, which can be helpful if they are tight. It also compresses the disks at their front and stretches them at their back, which can be beneficial if done cautiously. However, this flexion can aggravate existing problems or do damage if the structures in the lumbar area are fragile.

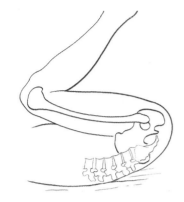

2 • *Extension*

When we bring our legs back toward the floor (beyond the tipping point), the muscles that contract to hold the legs up (primarily the psoas, iliacus, sartorius, rectus femoris, and tensor facsia latae) pull the pelvis into anteversion—an action that requires an equivalent contraction of the abdominals. If we don't prevent this anteversion, the lumbar spine is pulled into extension. This contraction creates strong compression of the vertebrae and the intervertebral disks at the back.

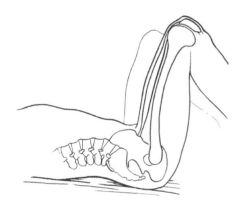

3 • *Stability*

If the pelvis isn't stabilized when we do various leg lifts, it's going to move alternately before and beyond the tipping point, squeezing the disks to the front and then to the back, which can put them under a great deal of stress. When adding leg beats (alternately crossing your ankles one over the other while your legs are lifted), it's very important to keep the pelvis fixed. Modify the range of motion depending on pelvic stability.

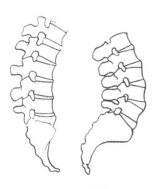

In leg lifts, the combination of the movement and compression is hard on the disks.

Protecting the Lumbar Spine

Precautions

It's absolutely imperative that we stabilize the pelvis during leg lifts. The pelvis shouldn't retrovert when we bring our legs into flexion; this requires the back muscles to work (see page 29). The pelvis shouldn't antevert when we bring our legs back to the floor; this requires the abominals to work (primarily the rectus abdominis). Yet for someone who has weak abdominals, it's not only impossible to keep the pelvis stable, it's often even difficult to feel when the pelvis is moving.

Stabilizing the Pelvis

To stabilize your pelvis, you can place your hands, palm down, under the lumbar spine. Your hands will prevent the lower back from rounding.

You can also work with just one leg (bent or straight).

Bend the supporting leg at the knee and place the foot on the floor. The pressure of the foot on the floor will inhibit the arching of your lower back. With your free leg, you can perform leg lifts of varying degrees of difficulty.

While performing the exercise, you can make it progressively more difficult by:

- Releasing the pressure on your supporting foot, letting the abdominals take over the work
- Avoiding letting your lower back touch the hand that you've placed under it, letting the back muscles take over the work

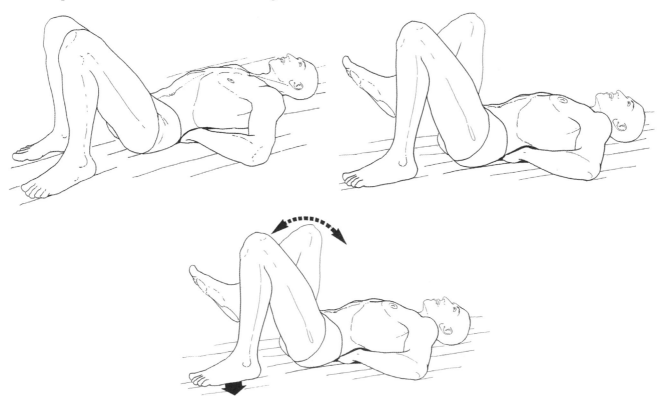

PUSH-UPS

+ **The Basic Push-up**
+ **How Push-ups Work the Abs**
+ **Push-ups Can Endanger the Perineum**
+ **Push-ups Can Endanger the Lumbar Spine**
+ **Protecting the Lumbar Spine**

The Basic Push-up

When we do a push-up, the only parts of the body that touch the floor are the toes and the palms.

We try not to let the lower back sag. We also try not to bend at the hip (sticking the butt out).

The exercise consists of bending and then straightening the arms while keeping the body in a plank position.

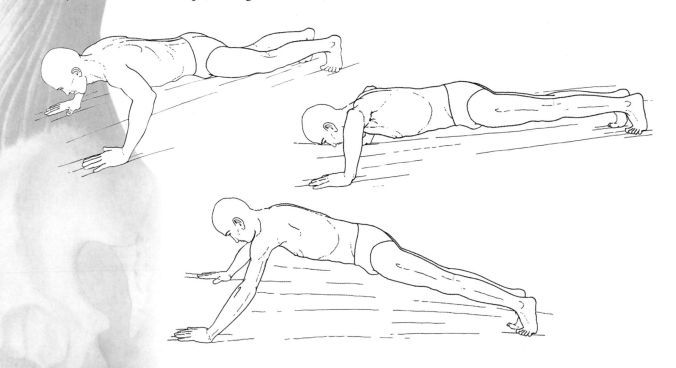

How Push-ups Work the Abs

We start by finding a balance between our hands and the feet, with our legs and trunk between the areas of support.

When our muscles are not well developed, the spine tends to move into a big arch in plank position and the pelvis into anteversion. The abdominals are forced to contract to prevent these two actions:

- They keep the spine from arching.
- They also keep the pelvis aligned.

They work in a static or isometric contraction.

The hips, knees, and ankles tend to bend. To prevent these areas from flexing, we are forced to contract the extensors in all of these areas at the same time.

The belly, which is now facing downward, tends to stick out. We must contract the abdominals in "visceral" mode to keep the belly pulled in.

During the push-up itself, the elbows flex and extend, which calls on the extensors of the elbows. They work to extend the arms when we are pressing up and to brake the flexion when we are lowering ourselves toward the floor.

When we do push-ups, the abdominals work statically, in other words, without any movement of the trunk. If we can keep the pelvis stable, the exercise, unlike crunches, can be powerful without endangering the skeleton. Push-ups can, however, put excessive pressure on the wrists if the position is held too long. In addition, the work of the abdominals is strictly isometric, which means that it does not improve blood flow in the muscles.

Push-ups Can Endanger the Perineum

On the face of it, push-ups don't seem to affect the perineum at all. However, push-ups are tough for the upper body, and we tend to close the glottis in an effort to keep the rib cage open. If the glottis is closed and we make a pushing effort against it, this puts pressure on the perineum (see page 32).

The pressure on the perineum can be caused:

- Directly, by the diaphragm moving toward the perineum

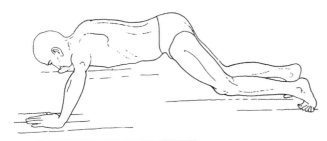

When we are new to push-ups the spine tends to arch; hips, knees, and ankles bend; and the belly tends to protrude in plank position.

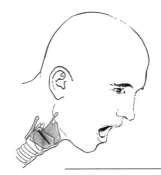

We tend to close the glottis when doing push-ups.

- Indirectly, by an ascending contraction of the abdominals sending pressure toward the glottis; if the glottis is closed, the pressure then descends toward the perineum

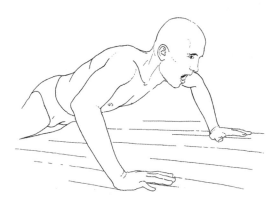

When we do push-ups, therefore, it's important to keep breathing and, above all, to avoid "pushing" with the glottis closed.

Push-ups Can Endanger the Lumbar Spine

Swayback and Lumbar Disk Compression
If our abdominals aren't strong enough, we can't maintain our trunk in good alignment when doing push-ups. The lumbar spine then usually goes into lordosis (swayback).

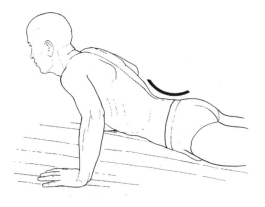

At the same time, we often let our belly bulge toward the floor.

Lordosis in and of itself isn't dangerous. However, in this position, with the abdominals in strong contraction trying to maintain the position of the trunk, the intervertebral disks are put under tremendous pressure.

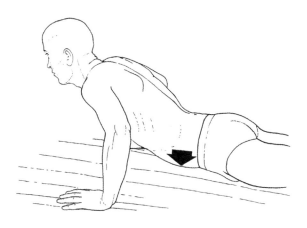

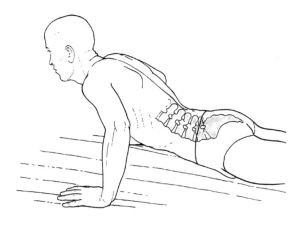

The combination of lordosis and compression can overtax the lumbar disks.

Protecting the Lumbar Spine

Precautions

If we can't align our trunk and legs without creating lordosis, it's better to lift our hips a bit toward the ceiling.

This posture is not ideal for push-ups, but it is a way to adapt the exercise for beginners. Here the abdominal muscles will function more to pull in the belly than to stabilize the pelvis.

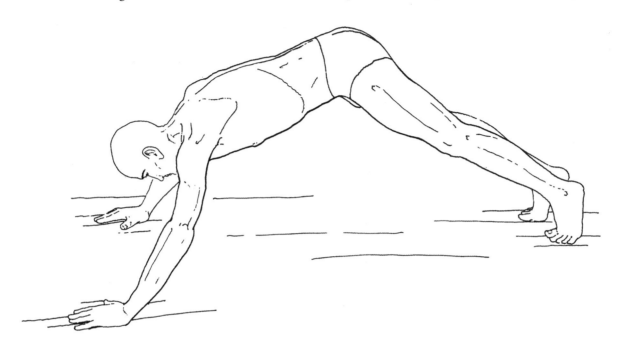

SUPINE TRUNK ROTATION

✦ **The Basic Rotation**

✦ **How Rotation Works the Abs**

✦ **Trunk Rotation Can Alternately Contract the Broad Muscles**

✦ **Trunk Rotation Can Endanger the Intervertebral Disks**

✦ **Protecting the Intervertebral Disks**

The Basic Rotation

1. Lie on your back, with your arms extended on each side.
2. Bring your legs in toward your chest, with your knees bent.
3. Drop your legs from one side to the other. Your trunk follows the movement, causing the vertebrae to rotate.

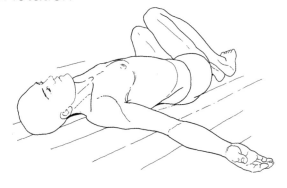

This exercise can be done with your legs bent or straight and raised or lowered. You can even place your feet on the floor.

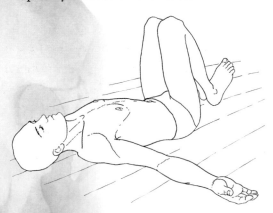

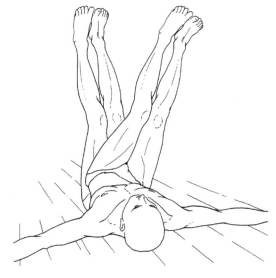

84

How Rotation Works the Abs

When we drop our legs toward the floor on one side, the pelvis is pulled into rotation toward that same side. The major factor in this movement is gravity (the weight of the legs).

The abdominals work to control the movement of the legs and the speed at which they fall toward the floor. However, above all, the abdominals that work in rotation are those broad muscles on the opposite side of the trunk, which contract to rotate the legs back up. The principal actors are the obliques.

In the rotation of the trunk, the abdominals move the trunk, not the legs. The legs are joined to the pelvis by the muscles of the hip.

Trunk Rotation Can Alternately Contract the Broad Muscles

The abdominals are as much in play when we lower our legs as when we lift them.

When we lower our legs, the abdominals act to control both the pelvis and the legs. We call this an eccentric contraction. Here, the muscles contract, but at the same time they stretch because the insertions of the muscles are moving away from each other.

When our intention is to bring our legs back to vertical, the opposite happens, and the same muscles actually cause the action. They contract to rotate the trunk back to the starting position. We call this a concentric contraction. In this kind of contraction, the muscle contracts and shortens because the insertion points are moving toward each other.

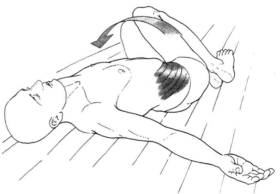

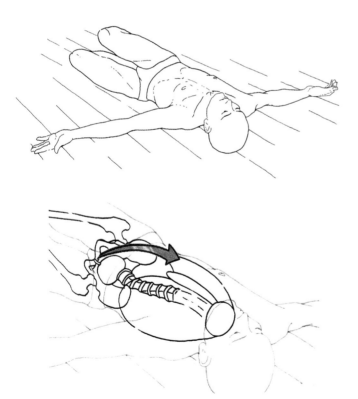

This stretching and shortening during contraction is an interesting way to work the muscle fibers, as it encourages blood flow and drainage (see page 50).

Trunk Rotation Can Endanger the Intervertebral Disks

Strong rotation torques the intervertebral disks. Strong contraction of the abdominals to hold the trunk or to initiate trunk rotation (when raising the legs) or brake trunk rotation (when lowering the legs) causes strong compression of the disks. The combination of strong torsion and strong compression can compromise the intervertebral disks, especially if they are already fragile.

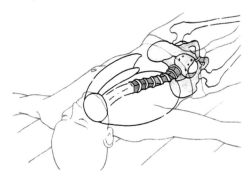

Protecting the Intervertebral Disks

We can reduce the intensity of the exercise:

- By working with our legs bent and our feet close to our pelvis; this reduces the size of the lever that is created by the legs
- By reducing the range of motion and limiting how far the legs fall toward the floor

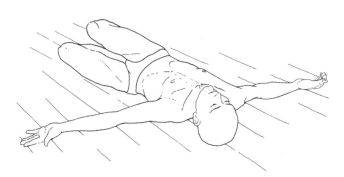

We can make sure that we stop our legs at the middle of the movement, when they are in line with gravity, and let our muscles rest.

We often do just the opposite, resting when our legs are closest to the floor and therefore the torsion/compression is at its maximum.

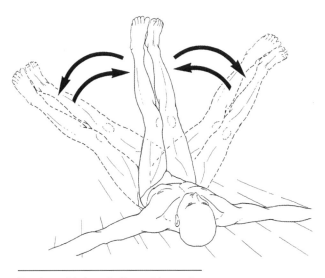

Resting with legs in line with gravity

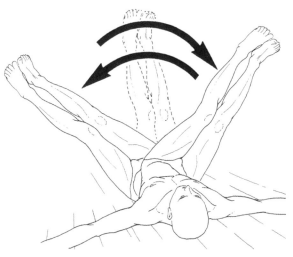

As the legs move closer to the floor, torsion and compression increase.

We can put our palms flat on the floor and use the pressure of our hands on the floor to help direct the movement. This pressure also solicits the back muscles, which assist in stabilizing the vertebrae during the movement.

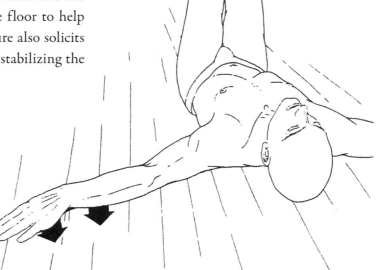

PULLING IN THE BELLY
ON A FORCEFUL EXHALATION

✦ **Engaging the Transversus Abdominis**

✦ **Engaging the Transversus Abdominis Narrows the Waist**

✦ **Forceful Exhalation Can Endanger the Perineum**

✦ **Forceful Exhalation Can Endanger the Linea Alba**

✦ **The Transversus Abdominis Can Work against Ascending Contraction of the Abdominals**

Engaging the Transversus Abdominis

When we do abdominal exercises, we often pull in our belly on a forceful exhalation. Sometimes the principal component of the exercise is simply to exhale through an open mouth with the glottis open as well.

A forceful exhalation through an open mouth is the most direct way to find the transversus abdominis. Why? By emptying the air from our lungs very rapidly in this way, we quickly come to the end of the exhalation and reach what is called the expiratory reserve volume (ERV).* This movement mobilizes the transversus abdominis.

> To find the transversus abdominis, we make a forceful and complete exhalation while pulling in our belly.

---

*See the book *Anatomy of Breathing,* by Blandine Calais-Germain (Seattle: Eastland Press, 2006).

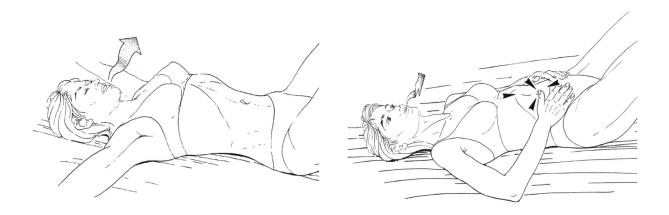

Engaging the Transversus Abdominis Narrows the Waist

An isolated contraction of the transversus abdominis will narrow the waist, but that's not really a benefit. The action of the transversus abdominis is limited predominantly to the area between the ribs and the pelvis, where the muscle's fibers are the longest and most numerous. A strong contraction of the transversus abdominis feels like a corset around the waist.

When we contract the transversus abdomi-

nis, we can't really actively direct the abdominal mass upward or downward. The viscera are simply pushed either above or below where the waist is squeezed. The abdominal mass that is pushed downward puts pressure on the perineum (see the following page). The abdominal mass that is pushed

The isolated contraction of the transversus abdominis also separates the linea alba (see page 37).

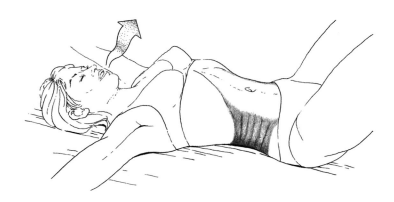

Forceful Exhalation Can Endanger the Perineum

The selective engagement of the transversus abdominis around or above the waist has some negative effects. In particular, when we exhale deeply while pulling in our belly, we create an hourglass effect. The waist narrows like a tube of toothpaste being squeezed in the middle, pushing the viscera upward and downward.

If the viscera are pushed upward, they do not affect the perineum. If they are pushed downward, though, they create pressure on the perineum. This pressure is not always desirable, especially if the perineum is not toned.

Abdominal exercises on their own create pressure on the perineum (such as when we roll up our trunk in a crunch; see pages 64–65). When we add a forceful exhalation, the strong contraction of the transversus abdominis creates additional pressure on the perineum.

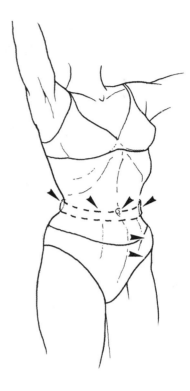

We can see how exhaling forcefully while pulling in our belly compromises the perineum. Even so, we do it, because it feels natural. That said, it is generally preferable to do crunches on an inhalation, with the ribs open, to reduce the pressure generated by the contraction of the transversus abdominis.

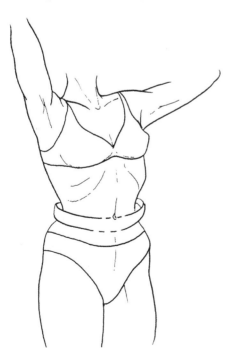

Forceful Exhalation Can Endanger the Linea Alba

The contractile part of the transversus abdominis is found not at the front of the body, but at the sides. The muscle therefore pulls in only the sides of the trunk. The transversus abdominis does indeed have fibers at the front of the belly, but they are noncontractile; they don't shorten. On the contrary, these fibers, forming the aponeuroses, are pulled on and put under tension by a contraction of the transversus abdominis.

There are two transversus abdominis muscles, one on each side of the body. Their aponeuroses meet in the midline of the abdomen, at the linea alba (see page 11). When contracted, the aponeurosis of each muscle is pulled toward the contractile part of the muscle. That is to say, the aponeuroses are pulled in opposite directions, stretching the linea alba. Normally the linea alba can withstand this action, because the interlacing of muscle fibers reinforces this area.

However, in certain cases the linea alba is overstretched—during pregnancy, for example, particularly in the last months (especially if the woman is pregnant with twins, or her pregnancy follows closely upon a previous one). After the birth, the fibers of the linea alba will slowly return to their original form, but even so, they can't tolerate severe traction.

For this reason, women should avoid specifically recruiting the transversus abdominis during pregnancy and after giving birth. People with hernias of the linea alba or the navel should also avoid recruiting this muscle. This group should therefore avoid pulling in the belly on an exhalation while exercising. They should preferably work the abs only on a costal inhalation.

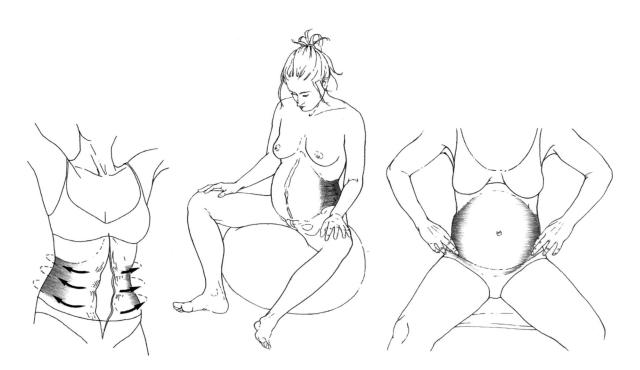

A contraction of the transversus abdominis stretches the linea alba.

Pregnant women should avoid recruiting the transversus abdominis.

The Transversus Abdominis Can Work against Ascending Contraction of the Abdominals

Some forms of abdominal work call for contracting the perineum and abdominals in an ascending fashion.* Most of us find it easy to keep the perineum contracted while we are contracting the lower abs.

of the transversus abdominis tends to pull in the waist and "cut the trunk in two" (see pages 14–15, 42–48, and 90).

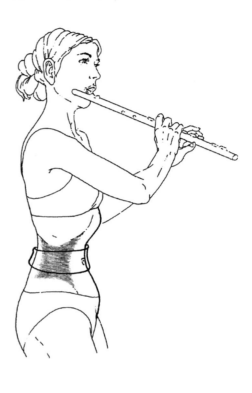

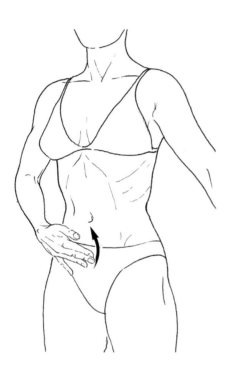

However, when we want to take the contractions further up the belly, we have a tendency to relax the perineum.

When the contraction of the abdominals from bottom to top reaches the level of the waist, it meets the horizontal fibers of the transversus abdominis. These fibers exert a strong force. We've seen how the contraction

Contraction of the transversus abdominis, which occurs naturally when we pull in the belly on a forced exhalation, pushes the viscera upward and downward. That downward pressure toward the perineum tends to make it relax.

If this is the case, we've inverted the desired muscle contraction order. Instead of coordinating the lift and contraction of the perineum with an ascending contraction of the abdominals, we've just contracted the abdominals and relaxed the perineum.

*See *The Female Pelvis: Anatomy & Exercises*, by Blandine Calais-Germain (Seattle: Eastland Press, 2003).

PART FOUR

Safe and Effective Exercises for Great Abs

- ✦ *The Six "No-Risk Abs" Principles*
- ✦ *Seven "No-Risk Abs" Preparatory Exercises*
- ✦ *Sixteen "No-Risk Abs" Exercises*

THE SIX "NO-RISK ABS" PRINCIPLES

+ Keep the Ribs Open No Matter How You're Breathing

+ Coordinate the Abs with the Perineum

+ Coordinate the Rectus Abdominis with the Transversus Abdominis

+ Coordinate the Obliques with the Transversus Abdominis

+ For Abs/Glute Work, Open the Front of the Hips

+ Coordinate the Abdominal and Back Muscles

On the following pages you will find a series of abdominal exercises that make up a part of the complete No-Risk Abs series. These exercises reflect the observations made in the preceding pages of this book, in particular pages 39–56.

These exercises are presented not as therapy, but as a means to improve body awareness and enhance training. They do not take pathologies into account. They can, however, be included in a therapy program and modified by a qualified professional to accommodate individual pathologies.

Any reader wishing to perform the exercises contained in these pages must be medically fit to participate in an exercise program. Some of these exercises may not be suitable for everyone; caution should be taken and modifications made for those suffering from diseases of the spine, rheumatological diseases, cancers, cardiovascular disease, or neurological or psychiatric disorders. In all of these cases the reader should seek the advice of the treating physician before beginning the exercises.

These also are not the only abdominal exercises that you can do. However, these exercises allow for a coordination of the breath that may be quite different from what you are used to when working the abdominals. The types of breathing proposed here, in particular the rib cage breathing, are meant to be done when performing the abdominal exercises. The reader should not infer that these types of breathing should be used all of the time. On the contrary, it is healthy to vary the way that you breathe when you exercise, as well as in daily life.*

Important Note

If you are not accustomed to exercising or are not a physical therapist or a teacher of a movement technique, it is indispensable to learn this series of exercises from a teacher trained in the No-Risk Abs technique.

---

*For more about breathing, please see the book *Anatomy of Breathing,* by Blandine Calais-Germain (Seattle: Eastland Press, 2006).

PRINCIPLE 1

Keep the Ribs Open
No Matter How You're Breathing

The first thing to remember is that there are many methods of breathing* and a number of ways that we can inhale and exhale. When doing abdominal exercises, we tend to do them in a way that causes our ribs to close. As a consequence, we breathe with the movement that closes the ribs, rather than consciously exercising the abdominals on an inhalation or exhalation.

We tend to inhale diaphragmatically, so that the diaphragm lowers and pushes the belly out. On the exhalation, we tend to close our ribs. In both cases, the consequences are the same: the belly expands, but there is a lot of downward pressure on the perineum—something it's best to avoid.

This is why, in many of the following exercises, the preferred breath is an inhalation to open the ribs at the moment that the abdominals tend to "close" the bones (at the moment that their action is in the "skeletal" mode). This opening of the ribs is easy to find on the inhalation, but difficult to find and maintain on the exhalation. We'll leave that to the experts. When you're doing the exercises, we propose that you open the ribs on the inhalation, when the abdominals are in "visceral" mode, and simply try to keep the ribs open on the exhalation, when you draw the belly in.

While doing abdominal exercises, we tend to repeatedly close the ribs. Before starting an exercise it's helpful to anticipate this closure of the ribs and try to work with them more open.

See preparatory exercises 1, "Mobilize the Ribs" (pages 102–3), and 2, "Tone the Muscles That Open the Ribs" (pages 103–4).

The preference is to breathe with the ribs open when the abdominals are the most active, whether on the inhalation (easier) or the exhalation (harder).

---

*See *Anatomy of Breathing,* by Blandine Calais-Germain (Seattle: Eastland Press, 2006).

PRINCIPLE 2

Coordinate the Abs and the Perineum

The abdominals directly influence the state of the perineum. Working the abdominals in a less than ideal way can damage the perineum. Conversely, coordinating the work of the abs and perineum can have a beneficial effect on the latter.

How can the abdominals damage the perineum?

• Dropping and closing the ribs pushes the organs downward toward the pelvis and generates pressure in the lower abdominal cavity.

• Flexing the spine from the head to the tailbone also pushes the organs downward toward the pelvis. This too creates pressure in the perineum, albeit less than closing the ribs creates.

• When the contraction of the abdominals themselves in the "visceral" mode pushes the organs downward, they are directly responsible for pressure on the perineum. Sometimes this is intentional, as during defecation, urination, and childbirth. But outside of these situations, this pushing is most often undesirable.

How do we protect the perineum when doing abdominal exercises?

• Give the perineum a "wake-up call" by doing a few perineum exercises before each session of abs work.

• Contract the perineum every time a movement pushes the organs downward. In other words, when the abdominals are working in "skeletal" mode, contract the perineum to help it withstand the pressure.

• Reduce the pressure on the perineum by keeping the ribs open whenever the abdominal mass is being pushed toward the pelvis.

It is imperative to protect the perineum when doing abdominal exercises.
See preparatory exercise 3, "Coordinate the Abs and the Perineum" (pages 104–5).

PRINCIPLE 3

Coordinate the Rectus Abdominis and Transversus Abdominis

We've seen how the transversus abdominis, the dominant muscle of the waist, wraps around the midsection to give us that "hourglass" shape. To more completely pull in the belly, we need to coordinate the action of the transversus abdominis with the action of the other abdominal muscles. Let's look first at the rectus abdominis.

If we don't want to send the contents of the abdominal cavity heading southward, we must support the lower belly by activating the lowest part of the rectus abdominis. In the exercises that follow, it is this action of the rectus abdominis that we're looking for each time we do an abdominal contraction in the "visceral" mode.

Why coordinate the action of the transversus abdominis and the rectus abdominis?

The lower fibers of the rectus abdominis are the only ones in the front of the abdomen that lift the contents of the abdominal cavity away from the perineum. In addition, the rectus is the only abdominal muscle that doesn't work in a way that separates the linea alba (see page 37).

See preparatory exercise 4, "Coordinate the Rectus Abdominis with the Transversus Abdominis" (pages 105–6).

PRINCIPLE 4

Coordinate the Obliques and Transversus Abdominis

We now know how the transversus abdominis dominates and encircles the waist like a corset. But it can't pull in the belly completely by itself. For this we need to solicit the other abdominal muscles as well. Let's look now at the obliques.

If we want to contract the transversus abdominis without pushing the contents of the abdominal cavity toward the lower belly, we need to counteract the downward push by contracting the lower fibers of the obliques. In the exercises that follow, we'll look to find this co-contraction whenever we contract the abdominals in "visceral" mode.

Like the rectus abdominis, the lower fibers of the obliques lift the contents of the abdomen away from the perineum, but in a more lateral manner. For this reason it's important to coordinate the obliques with the transversus abdominis.

See preparatory exercise 5, "Coordinate the Obliques with the Transversus Abdominis" (page 106).

PRINCIPLE 5

For Abs/Glute Work, Open the Front of the Hips

Certain exercises are designed to work the abs and the glutes at the same time. Both of these muscle groups place the pelvis in retroversion—a tuck. Therefore, these exercises strongly retrovert the pelvis.

The hip joint is not always ready for the pelvis to retrovert. Often the muscles and ligaments in the front of the hip are tight, which places the joint in a bit of flexion. Sitting for long periods of time is often the cause of this tightness. Strengthening the glutes in this situation compresses the hip joint and puts the cartilage there under tension as well. For this reason, we must open the front of the hip before doing abdominal or glute work.

Similarly, if the front of the hip is in a bit of flexion, when we stand up, we find that our pelvis is pulled into anteversion, creating excessive curve in the lower back. Here too, we need to free up what are essentially "brakes" in the front of the hip before we reinforce the abs and glutes, which pull the pelvis into retroversion.

Before working the abs and the glutes, it's important to relax the ligaments and muscles at the front of the hip.

See preparatory exercise 6, "Open the Front of the Hips" (page 107).

PRINCIPLE 6

Coordinate the Abdominal and Back Muscles

The abdominals tuck (retrovert) the pelvis and take the natural lordotic curve out of the spine. Though you might look to do this deliberately, to elongate the spine, it is not the normal position of the spine.

This is why you should keep a small curve in the lumbar region when you contract the abs. To keep this position, the back muscles must contract concurrently (see page 29). The abdominal and back muscles work in opposition on the lumbar spine, thereby maintaining equilibrium and keeping the lower back in a position that is neither excessively arched nor tucked.

When doing abdominal exercises it is important to keep the pelvis and back in balance, maintaining the natural lordotic curve of the spine. This action requires not just the abdominals but other muscles as well, and in particular the muscles at the back of the pelvis and the spine.

See preparatory exercise 7, "Coordinate the Abdominal and Back Muscles" (pages 107–8).

SEVEN "NO-RISK ABS" PREPARATORY EXERCISES

✦ Mobilize the Ribs

✦ Tone the Muscles That Open the Ribs

✦ Coordinate the Abs with the Perineum

✦ Coordinate the Rectus Abdominis with the Transversus Abdominis

✦ Coordinate the Obliques with the Transversus Abdominis

✦ Open the Front of the Hips

✦ Coordinate the Abdominal and Back Muscles

Preparatory Exercise I

Mobilize the Ribs

Part I

1. Lie on your back with your knees bent and your feet flat on the floor.
2. Slide your arms along the floor, drawing an arc on each side of your trunk.
3. Return to the starting position.
4. Feel how the movement opens the ribs, and allow this movement to happen.
   Feel:
   • The opening of the ribs and the rising of the sternum as the arms open
   • The return of the ribs as the arms return to the starting position

Repeat this exercise several times, slowly.

Part 2

1. Make the same movement with one arm.
2. When the arm gets to the level of your head, let your thorax follow naturally the movement of the arm.
3. Notice that the ribs open more on the side of the arm that's lifting.
4. Return to the starting position.
5. Repeat the movement on the other side.

Preparatory Exercise 2

Tone the Muscles That Open the Ribs

Part 1a

The ribs have a tendency to close, so it's necessary to work the muscles of inhalation to keep the ribs open and separated.

1. Lie on your back. Inhale deeply, opening the ribs to the sides as if you were trying to make the rib cage wider.
2. Exhale, and let the ribs return to their original position.
3. Take several normal breaths.

Part 1b

1. Start as in part 1a, but after taking a deep inhalation, instead of exhaling immediately, hold your breath for a moment, as if in suspension.
2. Then try to inhale a bit more and hold your breath again for a few seconds, before blowing the air out.
3. Take several normal breaths.

Repeat this process several times. This exercise works the muscles of inhalation, principally the serratus anterior.

Part 1c

Stand up, and repeat part 1b in this position.

Part 2a

Because the sternum tends to drop, it's necessary to work the muscles of inhalation to keep it lifted and forward.

1. Lie on your back. Inhale deeply, raising the sternum as if you wanted to make the thorax "deeper." While making this movement, try not to let your shoulder blades pull toward each other.
2. Exhale, and let the sternum fall.
3. Take several normal breaths.

Part 2b

1. Start as in part 2a, but just after taking a deep inhalation, instead of exhaling immediately, hold your breath for a moment, as if in suspension.
2. Then try to inhale a bit more, and hold your rib cage in that position, with the sternum raised, for a few seconds before blowing the air out.
3. Take several normal breaths.

Repeat this process several times. Among the muscles of inhalation, this series works the pectorals.

Part 2c

Stand up, and repeat part 2b in this position.

Preparatory Exercise 3

Coordinate the Abs with the Perineum

Part 1

1. Lie on your back, with your knees bent and feet flat on the floor.
2. Contract and relax the perineum. If you have never practiced this, you can, for example, contract-relax the sphincter of the anus, or contract-relax the area between the sitz bones by imagining that you are bringing them closer together.

Repeat this contraction and relaxation several times.

Part 2

1. Contract the perineum.
2. With the perineum still contracted, contract the lower abdominals as well, without letting the contraction rise toward the navel.

Practice this action several times—perineum first, then the lower abs. Don't allow the contraction to rise up to the waist, and don't relax the perineum as you contract the abdominals.

Part 3

1. Contract the perineum.
2. With the perineum still contracted, contract the lower abdominals. Now allow the contraction to move a bit higher up the abdominals, toward the navel.

Be sure to remember this important point: don't relax the perineum as you contract the abdominals.

Preparatory Exercise 4

Coordinate the Rectus Abdominis with the Transversus Abdominis

Part 1

1. Lie on your back, with your knees bent and feet flat on the floor.
2. Contract the portion of the rectus abdominis that lies at the front of the lower belly.
3. Relax.

Repeat this process several times.

Part 2

1. Contract the rectus abdominis progressively from the pubic bone to the navel, that is to say, from low to high.
2. Relax.

Repeat this process a dozen times. This is a very important step, as it guides the visceral mass from low to high.

Part 3

1. Again, contract the rectus abdominis progressively from the pubic bone to the navel. This time, when you reach the top of this progressive contraction,

contract the transversus abdominis as well, which should give you the sensation of narrowing the waist.

2. Relax.

Be sure to remember this important point: don't release the contraction of the rectus abdominis as you contract the transversus abdominis.

Preparatory Exercise 5

Coordinate the Obliques with the Transversus Abdominis

Part 1

1. Lie on your back, with your knees bent and feet flat on the floor.
2. Progressively contract the external obliques at the sides of the waist, while tracing the direction of their fibers from the pelvis to the ribs with your fingers.
3. Relax.

Repeat this process several times.

Part 2

1. Trace the path of the inguinal ligament with your fingers, which will cause an activation of the internal obliques, so that you know what area is put under tension when the lower part of the obliques is engaged.
2. Relax.

Repeat this process several times.

Part 3

1. Contract the obliques.
2. Now, with the obliques still contracted, contract the upper regions of the rectus abdominis and the transversus abdominis. This will give you the feeling of narrowing the waist.
3. Aim to keep the feeling of drawing in the lower belly.

Repeat this process a dozen or so times, so that you can memorize the feeling before starting abdominal exercises.

Preparatory Exercise 6

Open the Front of the Hips

Part 1

1. Lie on your stomach.
2. Bend your right knee, and grasp your right foot with a hand (right or left).
3. Feel how the right side of the pelvis is anteverted and the pubic bone has lifted off the floor.

Part 2

1. While holding your foot, try to place the pelvis and the public bone back on the floor, retroverting the pelvis.
2. Feel how this movement stretches the front of the hip.
3. Hold this position for several seconds, staying within a limit that is comfortable for your hip.
4. Relax.

Repeat parts 1 and 2 several times, and play with your breathing pattern, either on the inhalation (to open) or the exhalation (to relax).

Part 3

Repeat the entire exercise on the left side.

Preparatory Exercise 7

Coordinate the Abdominal and Back Muscles

This preparation can be practiced lying down or standing, depending on the choice of exercises that will follow.

Part 1a

1. Lie on your back, with your knees bent and feet flat on the floor.
2. Put a hand under the lumbar region, keeping your hand open. Raise your lower back just enough so your hand slides beneath you easily. The back muscles are at work here.

Part 1b

1. Contract the abdominals while keeping the lower back in this position. Feel how contracting the abdominals tends to send the pelvis into retroversion and pulls the lower back toward the floor.
2. Maintain the contraction of the back muscles to prevent this retroversion.

Repeat this process several times.

Part 2a

1. Stand with your knees slightly bent.
2. Put one hand behind the lumbar region, keeping your hand open.
3. Arch your lumbar spine slightly, while at the same time trying to stand taller and get as vertical as possible. This is the work of the back muscles, chiefly the deep back muscles.

Part 2b

1. Contract the abdominals while maintaining the back in this position. Feel how the contraction of the abdominals tends to pull the pelvis into retroversion and flatten the lordotic curve of the lower back.
2. Maintain the contraction of the back muscles to inhibit the retroverting action of the abdominals.

SIXTEEN "NO-RISK ABS" EXERCISES

✦ **Alternately Stretch and Contract the Abdominals**

1. Stretching the Rectus Abdominis
2. Contracting the Rectus Abdominis
3. Stretching the Internal Obliques
4. Contracting the Internal Obliques
5. Stretching the External Obliques
6. Contracting the External Obliques

✦ **Contract the Abdominals and Glutes**

7. Using Arm Movement to Contract the Obliques
8. Using Leg Movement to Contract the Obliques
9. Using Leg and Arm Movement to Contract the Obliques

✦ **Coordinate the Abdominals**

10. The Little Airplane

✦ **The Drawback Lunge**

11. Stretching the Rectus Abdominis with the Drawback Lunge
12. Contracting the Rectus Abdominis with the Drawback Lunge

✦ **The Turning Lunge**

13. Stretching the Obliques with the Turning Lunge
14. Contracting the Obliques with the Turning Lunge

✦ **The Side Lunge**

15. Stretching the Obliques with the Side Lunge
16. Contracting the Obliques with the Side Lunge

Alternately Stretch and Contract the Abdominals

Exercise I

Stretching the Rectus Abdominis

Lie on your back with your arms at your sides, knees bent, and feet flat on the floor. Cross your hands on your chest.

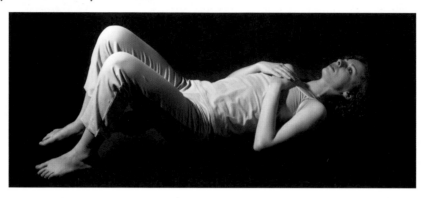

Stretch the Upper Part of the Rectus Abdominis ("Cross Lift")

1. With your hands crossed, reach your arms above your head, passing them over the front of your body (not to the sides).
2. Feel how this movement lifts the ribs and the sternum. Feel also how the upper part of the rectus abdominis stretches.
3. Return to the starting position.
4. Raise your arms again, while taking a deep inhalation into the ribs.
5. Return to the starting position.

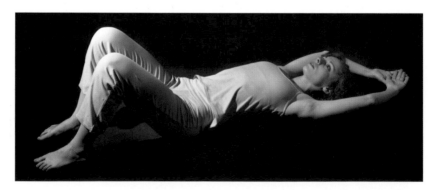

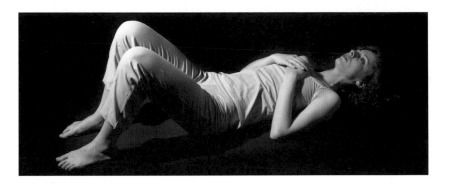

Stretch the Lower Part of the Rectus Abdominis ("Lengthen Arch")

1. Extend your legs, until they rest flat on the floor.
2. Feel how this movement pulls the pelvis into anteversion (i.e., an arch). Feel how this anteversion stretches the lower part of the rectus abdominis.
3. Return to the starting position.

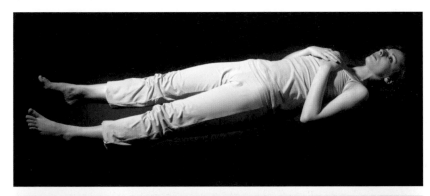

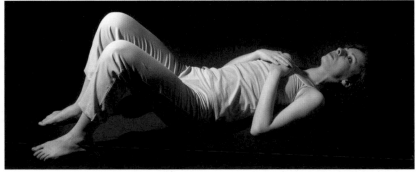

Exercise 1: Stretching the Rectus Abdominis

4. Extend your legs again, while taking a deep inhalation into the ribs.

5. Return to the starting position.

Stretch the Whole Rectus Abdominis ("Lift/Lengthen")

1. Raise your arms and extend your legs at the same time.

2. Feel how this movement stretches both the upper and lower reaches of the rectus abdominis.

3. Let the lumbar region arch, without trying to control it.

4. Return to the starting position.

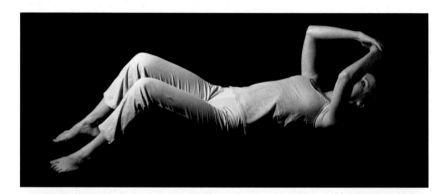

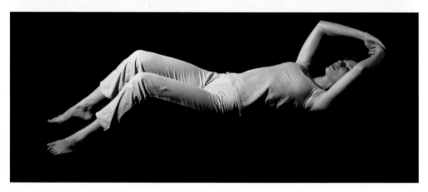

Alternately Stretch and Contract the Abdominals

5. Do the movement again, while taking a deep inhalation into the ribs that allows the sternum to rise.

6. Return to the starting position.

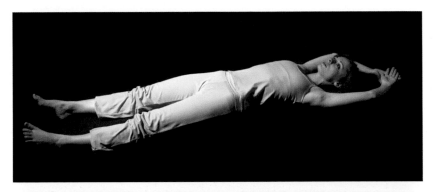

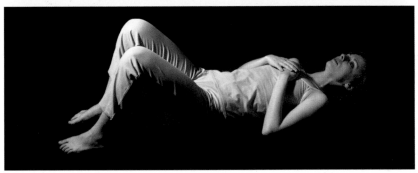

Exercise 2

Contracting the Rectus Abdominis

Lie on your back with your legs extended and your arms stretched over your head, with your hands crossed.

Contract the Rectus Abdominis in "Visceral" Mode ("Pull In")

1. Exhaling, contract the rectus abdominis as if you were trying to draw the pubic bone to the sternum, and the sternum toward the public bone, but without moving any of the bones. Don't press your lower back into the floor, and above all, don't pull your ribs down.
2. Return to the starting position.

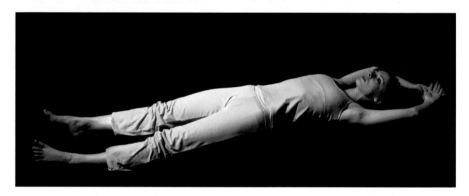

Contract the Rectus Abdominis in "Skeletal" Mode ("Knee")

1. Contract the rectus abdominis as described in the "Pull In" part of exercise 2.
2. Inhaling into the ribs, bring one leg toward your stomach, with the knee bent.
3. Exhaling, stretch the leg back out along the floor.
4. Relax as you inhale and exhale.
5. Repeat the "Knee" series with the other leg.
6. Now, inhaling, draw both legs in toward your stomach with the knees bent.
7. Exhaling, stretch both legs back out along the floor.
8. Relax as you inhale and exhale.

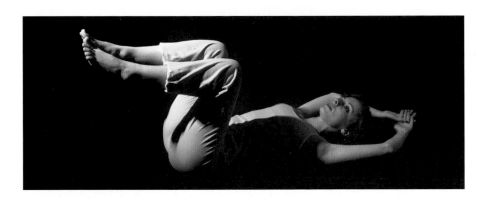

Contract the Rectus Abdominis in Static "Skeletal" Mode ("Chin")

1. Contract the rectus abdominis as described in the "Pull In" part of exercise 2.
2. Inhaling into the ribs, lift your head, bringing your chin toward your chest.
3. Exhaling, let your head back down.
4. Relax as you inhale and exhale.
5. Repeat the "Chin" series one more time.

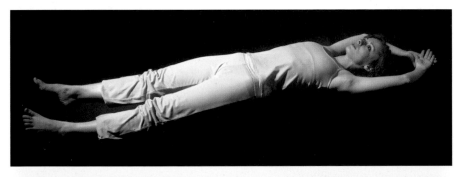

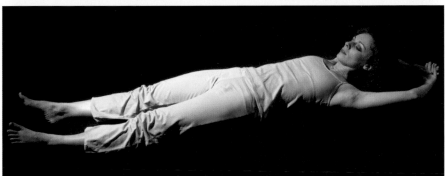

Exercise 2: Contracting the Rectus Abdominis

Contract the Rectus Abdominis More Intensely in Static "Skeletal" Mode ("Arms")

1. Contract the rectus abdominis as described in the "Pull In" part of exercise 2.
2. Inhaling into the ribs, lift your head and bring your arms toward the ceiling.
3. Exhaling, bring your head and arms back down.
4. Relax as you inhale and exhale.
5. Repeat the "Arms" series one more time.

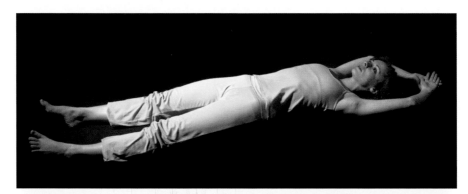

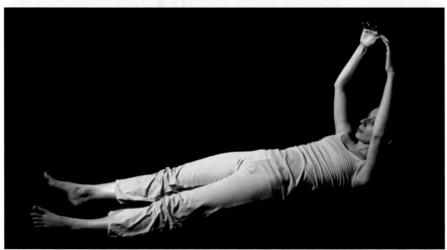

Alternately Stretch and Contract the Abdominals

Contract the Rectus Abdominis Most Intensely in Static "Skeletal" Mode ("Everything Lifted")

1. Contract the rectus abdominis as described in the "Pull In" part of exercise 2.
2. Inhaling into the ribs, lift your legs, head, and arms at the same time.
3. Exhaling, bring your legs, head, and arms back down.
4. Relax as you inhale and exhale.
5. Repeat the "Everything Lifted" series one more time.

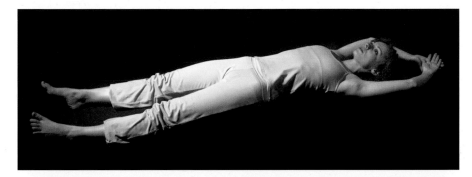

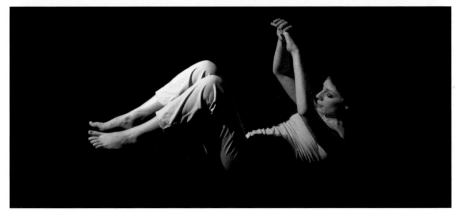

Exercise 3

Stretching the Internal Obliques

Lie on your back with your arms at your sides and legs flat on the floor.

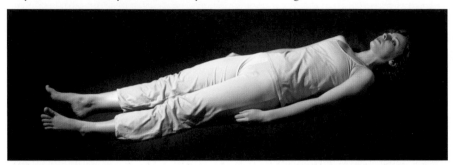

Stretch the Upper Part of the Right Internal Oblique ("Cross/Lift")

1. Bring your right arm across your chest, reaching on a diagonal to the upper left side of your body.
2. Feel how this movement stretches the top of the right internal oblique.
3. Return to the starting position.
4. Inhaling into the ribs, repeat the same movement, reaching with your right arm on a diagonal to the upper left side of your body.
5. Exhaling, return to the starting position.

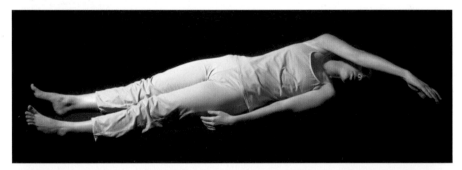

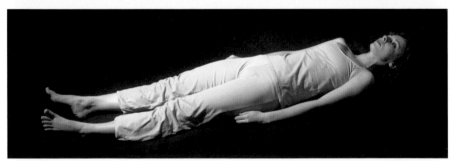

Alternately Stretch and Contract the Abdominals

*Fix the Lower Part of the Right Internal Oblique to Stretch the
Entire Muscle ("Cross/Turn")*

1. Still lying on your back, with your arms at your sides and legs flat on the floor, open your right leg on a diagonal along the floor, rotating the leg toward the outside from the hip.
2. Feel how this movement turns the pelvis slightly to the same side. Just let it turn.
3. Keeping your right leg in this position, repeat the first part of exercise 3 ("Cross/Lift"), reaching with your right arm on a diagonal to the upper left side of your body.

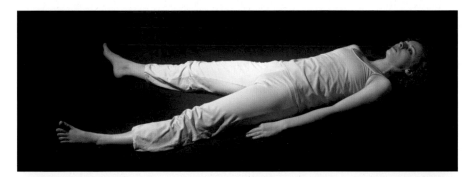

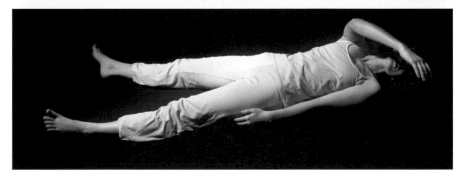

4. Feel how the rotation of the trunk now stretches the entire right internal oblique.

5. Return to the starting position.

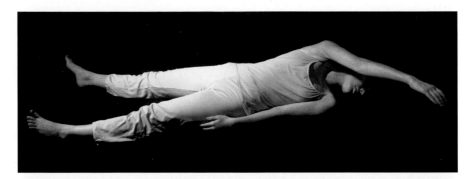

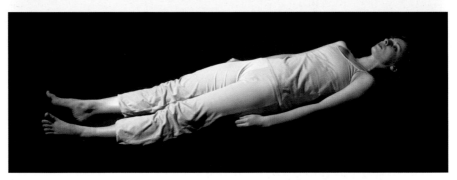

6. Inhaling into the ribs, repeat the same movements with your right leg and right arm.

7. Exhaling, return to the starting position.

Repeat the Series on the Left Side

1. Reaching your left arm across your body, perform the "Cross/Lift" part of the exercise to stretch the upper part of the left internal oblique.

2. Fixing your left leg and reaching with your left arm, perform the "Cross/Turn" part of the exercise to stretch the entire left internal oblique.

Alternately Stretch and Contract the Abdominals

Alternate Stretches of the Internal Obliques

1. Perform the "Cross/Turn" part of exercise 3 on one side and then the other to alternate stretching and contracting the two internal obliques.

2. Relax as you inhale and exhale.

3. Repeat the series one more time.

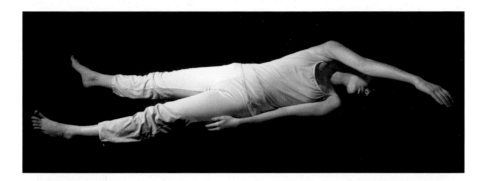

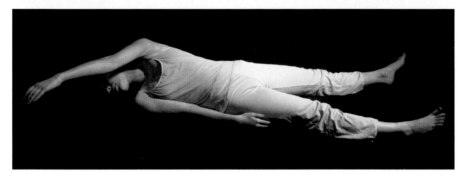

Exercise 4

Contracting the Internal Obliques

Lie on your back with your arms at your sides and legs flat on the floor.

Contract the Right Internal Oblique in "Visceral" Mode ("Cross/Turn/Pull In")

1. Inhaling into the ribs, perform the stretch described in the "Cross/Turn" part of exercise 3, reaching with your right arm on a diagonal to the upper left side of your body, and opening your right leg on a diagonal along the floor, rotating the leg to the outside from the hip.

2. Exhaling, contract the right internal oblique by bringing your right shoulder blade down to the floor while trying to lift the right side of the pelvis from the floor. Don't allow the exhalation to initiate the movement or lower ribs. Your belly should pull in, and pressure on the perineum will decrease.

3. Return to the starting position.

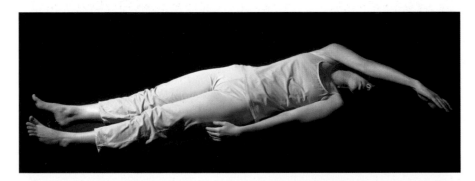

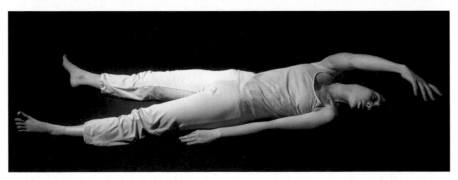

Alternately Stretch and Contract the Abdominals

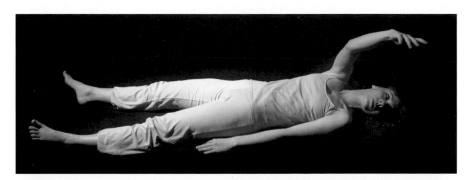

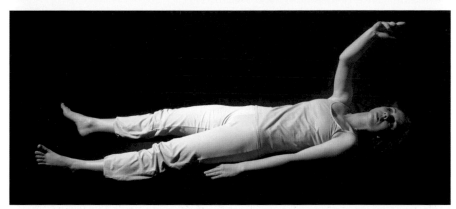

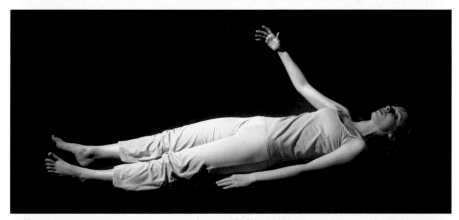

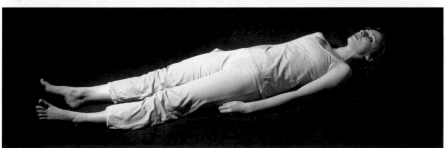

Exercise 4: Contracting the Internal Obliques

Contract the Right Internal Oblique in "Skeletal" Mode ("Return")

1. Get into the stretch/contract position described in the first part of exercise 4 ("Cross/Turn/Pull In").
2. Lift your head while turning it slightly to the left. Now, inhaling into the ribs, draw your right shoulder blade toward the floor, while bringing your head back to the center and drawing a large arc toward the ceiling with your right arm. Bring the arm back along your side.
3. Exhaling, place your head back on the floor.
4. Relax as you inhale and exhale.
5. Repeat the series one more time.

Repeat the Series on the Left Side

Repeat the first and second parts of exercise 4 ("Cross/Turn/Pull In" and "Return") on the opposite side, with your left arm and leg.

Alternate Contractions of the Internal Obliques

1. Practice the "Return" part of exercise 4 on one side and then the other to alternate stretching and contracting the two internal obliques.
2. Relax as you inhale and exhale.
3. Repeat the series one more time.

Alternately Stretch and Contract the Abdominals

Exercise 5

Stretching the External Obliques

Stretch the Lower Part of the Right External Oblique ("Leg Cross")

1. Lie on your back with your arms at your sides, your left leg extended on the floor, and your right leg bent at the knee, with its foot flat on the floor.
2. Cross your right leg over your left leg, stretching it as far as possible away from the pelvis.
3. Feel how this movement pulls the pelvis into rotation. Let the pelvis move. Feel how this movement stretches the lower part of the right external oblique.
4. Return to the starting position.
5. Inhaling into the ribs, make the same movement.
6. Exhaling, return to the starting position.

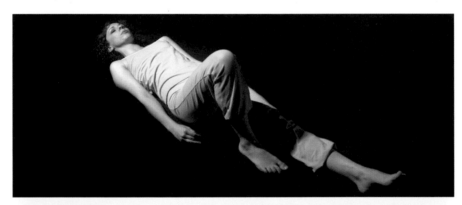

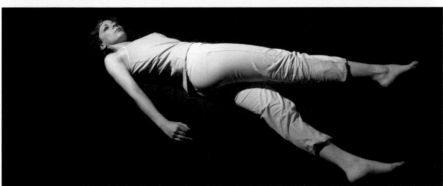

Stretch the Upper Part of the Right External Oblique ("Open Arms")

1. Now stretch your right arm above your head and away from your trunk.
2. Feel how this movement stretches the upper part of the right exterior oblique.
3. Return to the starting position.
4. Inhaling into your ribs, make the same movement.
5. Return to starting position.

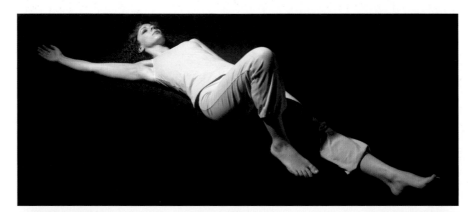

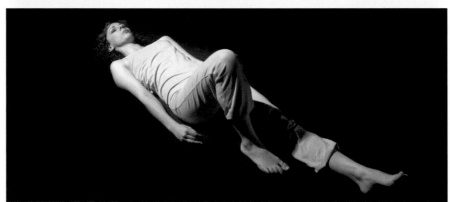

Stretch the Entire Right External Oblique ("Diagonal")

1. Perform the first and second parts of exercise 5 ("Leg Cross" and "Open Arms") at the same time. Stretch your right arm above your head and away from your trunk, while at the same time crossing your right leg over your left leg and stretching it away from the pelvis, to create a diagonal line from right hand to right foot.
2. Return to the starting position.
3. Inhaling into the right ribs, make the movement again.
4. Return to the starting position.

Alternately Stretch and Contract the Abdominals

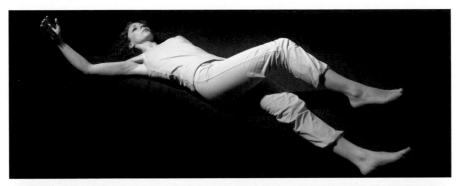

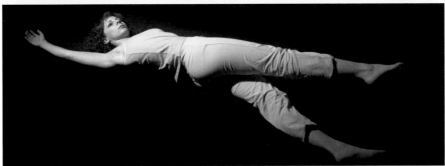

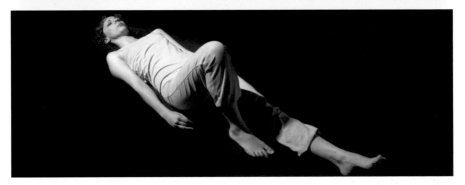

Repeat the Series on the Left Side

Repeat the "Leg Cross," "Open Arms," and "Diagonal" parts of exercise 5 on the left side.

Alternate Stretches of the External Obliques

1. Perform the "Diagonal" part of exercise 5 once on each side, alternately stretching the external obliques on each side.
2. Relax as you inhale and exhale.
3. Repeat on each side one more time.

Exercise 5: Stretching the External Obliques

Exercise 6

Contracting the External Obliques

Contract the Right External Oblique in "Visceral" Mode ("Diagonal/Pull In")

1. Perform the stretch described in the "Diagonal" part of exercise 5.
2. Exhaling, contract the right external oblique by bringing your pelvis and right shoulder blade back to the floor. Don't allow the exhalation to initiate the movement or lower the ribs. The belly will pull in and the pressure on the perineum will decrease.
3. Return to the starting position.

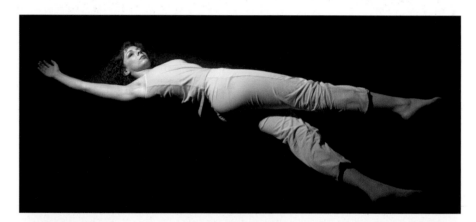

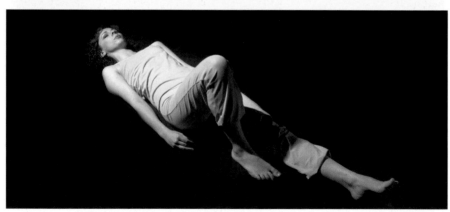

Contract the Right External Oblique
in "Skeletal" Mode ("Return")

1. Get into the stretched-out position described for the "Diagonal/Pull In" part of exercise 6, with the right external oblique contracted.
2. Exhaling, pull your pelvis down to the floor, letting the leg follow, drawing a large arc on the ceiling before you place the leg on the floor next to your left leg.
3. Relax as you inhale and exhale.
4. Repeat this movement one more time.

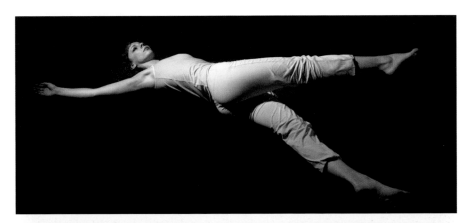

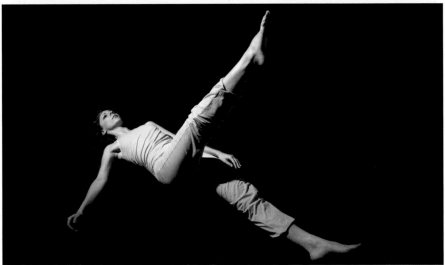

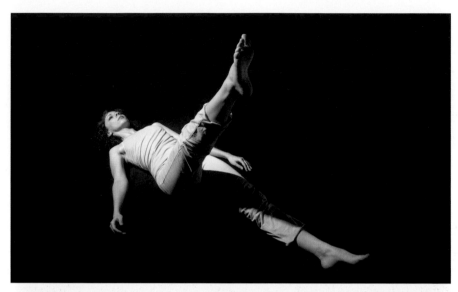

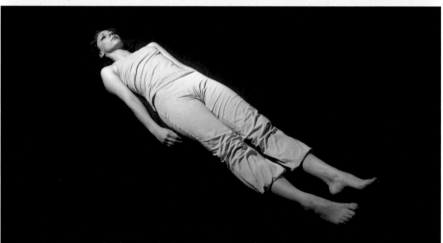

Repeat the Series on the Left Side

Repeat the "Diagonal/Pull In" and "Return" parts of exercise 6 on the opposite side.

Alternate Contractions of the External Obliques

1. Practice the "Return" part of exercise 5 on one side and then the other to alternate stretching and contracting the two external obliques.
2. Relax as you inhale and exhale.
3. Repeat the series one more time.

Alternately Stretch and Contract the Abdominals

Contract the Abdominals and Glutes

Exercise 7

Using Arm Movement to Contract the Obliques

1. Lie on your left side with your left arm extended in front of you, your left knee bent, and your right arm bent at the elbow.
2. Feel how pressing your arm into the floor stabilizes you and prevents your trunk from falling forward. Feel how pressing your left leg into the floor stabilizes your trunk and prevents it from falling backward.

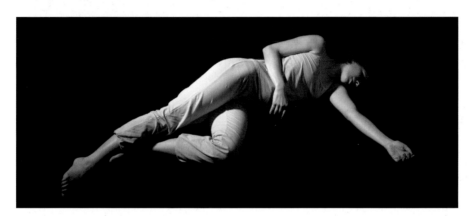

With the Arm in Front ("Lengthen")

1. Inhaling into the ribs, extend your right arm slowly to the front. The thorax tends to follow the arm in this movement. Feel the contraction of the internal oblique that keeps the thorax from falling forward.
2. Bring the arm back to its starting position.

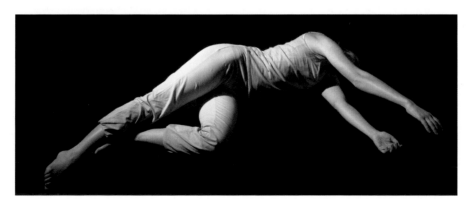

With the Arm Behind ("Return")

1. Inhaling into the ribs, extend your right arm slowly backward, more or less parallel to the floor. Here, the thorax wants to fall backward. Feel the contraction of the right external oblique that prevents this movement.
2. Bring the arm back to its starting position.

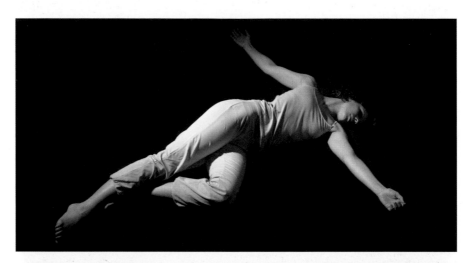

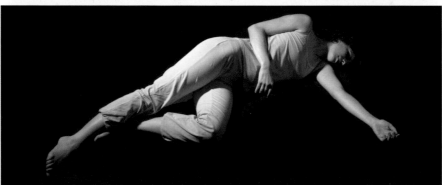

Contract the Abdominals and Glutes

Alternate Contractions of the Obliques

Alternate extending the arm to the front and the back, repeating these movements several times. Keep the ribs as stable as possible, reaching as far as possible each time.

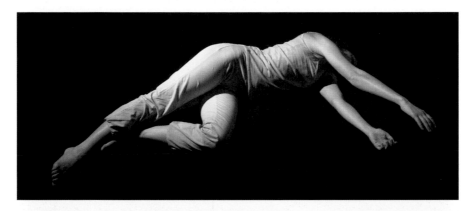

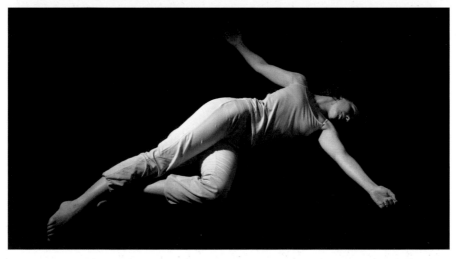

Intensify Contractions of the Obliques

1. Lie in the same position as in the preceding parts of exercise 7, but instead of placing your left arm in front of you, align it with your trunk, placing your head on your arm. This position requires greater stabilization from the abdominals.
2. Straighten your left leg, aligning it with your right leg. This requires even greater stabilization from the abdominals.
3. Perform the stretches described in the "Lengthen" and "Return" parts of exercise 7, alternating between them.

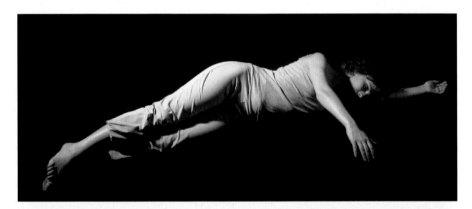

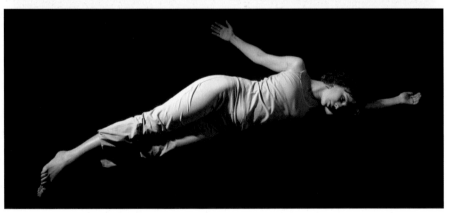

Repeat the Series Using the Left Arm

1. Perform the "Lengthen" and "Return" parts of exercise 7 using the left arm.
2. Intensify the contractions in your left obliques by straightening your right arm and right leg.
3. Then alternate between "Lengthen" and "Return" several times.

Contract the Abdominals and Glutes

Exercise 8

Using Leg Movement to Contract the Obliques

Leg to the Front ("Kick")

1. Lie on your left side with your left arm extended in front of you, your left knee bent, and your right arm bent at the elbow.
2. Bend your right leg, bringing your foot close to your pelvis.
3. Inhaling into the ribs, kick your right leg out in front of you. The pelvis tends to follow this movement of the leg. Feel the contraction of the right external oblique stabilizing the pelvis, keeping it from falling forward.
4. Return to the starting position.

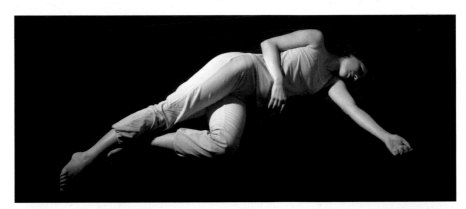

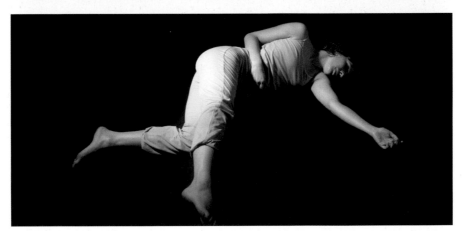

Leg to the Back ("Lengthen")

1. Bend your right leg again, bringing your foot close to your pelvis.
2. Inhaling into the ribs, extend your right leg backward, more or less parallel to the floor. Here, the pelvis tends to fall backward. Feel the contraction of the right internal oblique keeping the pelvis stable.

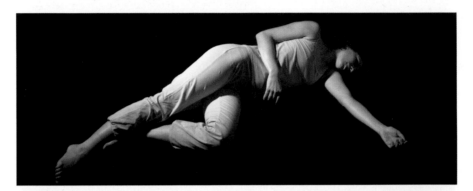

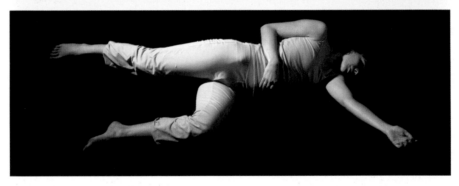

Link the Movements ("Balance")

Perform several kicks to the front and then several to the back, while keeping the pelvis stable. This alternates contractions of the internal and external obliques.

Contract the Abdominals and Glutes

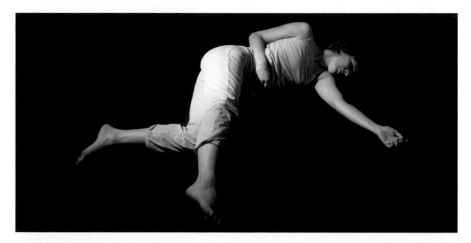

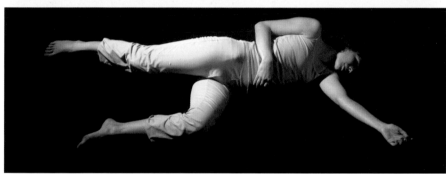

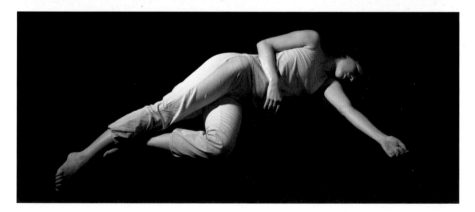

Repeat the Series on the Left Side

1. Perform the "Kick" and "Lengthen" parts of exercise 8 with the left leg.
2. Do the "Balance" part of exercise 8 with the left leg, performing several kicks to front and back while keeping the pelvis stable.

Exercise 8: Using Leg Movement to Contract the Obliques

Exercise 9

Using Leg and Arm Movement to Contract the Obliques

Combine the Movements to Stretch the Obliques ("Double Balance")

1. Lie in the same starting position as for exercises 7 and 8: on your left side with your left arm extended in front of you, your left knee bent, and your right arm bent at the elbow.

2. At the same time, perform the "Lengthen" movements of exercises 7 and 8, bringing your right arm forward and your right leg back.

3. When the arm and the leg are totally extended, feel how this diagonal reach stretches the internal oblique. Reach as far as you can with the arm and the leg to intensify the stretch.

4. Then move into the "Return" movement of exercise 7 and the "Kick" movement of exercise 8, extending your right arm backward and your right leg forward. Feel how this diagonal reach stretches the external oblique. Reach as far as you can with the arm and the leg to intensify the stretch.

5. Perform this series four times.

6. Repeat the series with your left arm and leg, transitioning to it by turning onto your back and other side without interrupting the movement.

*Connect the Movements to
Alternate Stretches and Contractions*

1. Now align your left arm with your trunk, placing your head on your arm. This position is quite intense and requires greater stabilization from the obliques.

2. Straighten your left leg, aligning it with your right leg. This too demands even greater stabilization from the obliques.

3. In this position, perform the "Double Balance" part of exercise 9.

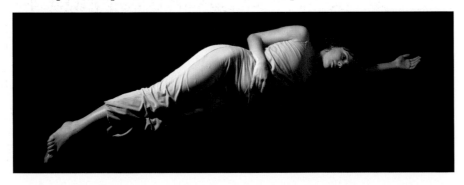

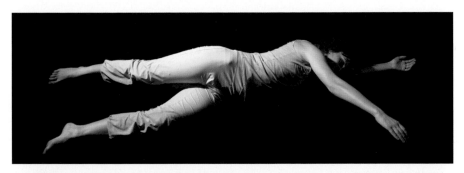

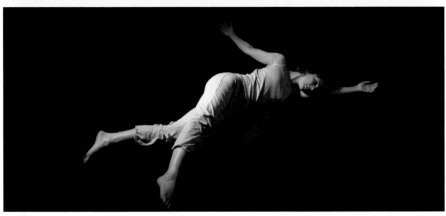

Connect the Movements with a Contraction of the Rectus Abdominis

Perform the movements of the preceding section ("Connect the Movements to Alternate Stretches and Contractions") again. Throughout the series keep your head off the ground to contract the rectus abdominus.

Exercise 9: Using Leg and Arm Movement to Contract the Obliques

Coordinate the Abdominals

Exercise 10

The Little Airplane

For this exercise you will need an inflatable ball, 20 centimeters (8 inches) in diameter, inflated to about half of its capacity. The exercise changes according to where you place the ball under the body.

"Lift Off"

1. Lie on your back, with your knees bent and feet flat on the floor. Place the ball under your sacrum.
2. Lift your feet off the floor. Immediately you will feel the rectus abdominis engage, first to stabilize the pelvis and keep it from going into anteversion, and then to bring the pelvis toward the belly as you bring your bent legs in.

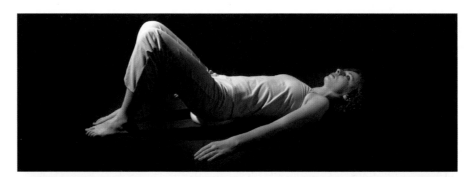

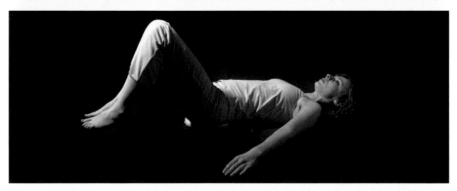

"Stabilization"

1. Keeping your feet raised, stabilize your body on the ball so that you aren't moving from side to side. It will help to push your hands into the floor. This works the muscles that press the arms back, in particular the latissimi dorsi in conjunction with the obliques and the rectus abdominis (in a static mode).

2. Next, lift both arms and try to stabilize your body using only the abdominals.

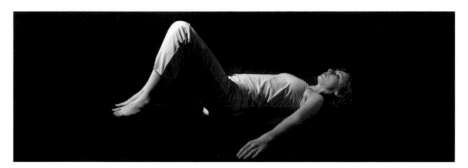

"Flight Events"

You can modify your position to affect and challenge your balance.

1. Extend your arms toward the ceiling. Slowly open both arms until they are almost parallel to the floor. Then bring them back to vertical. Repeat this movement with one arm and then the other.

2. Extend your legs toward the ceiling, and bring them close to your trunk. Slowly separate your legs, and then bring them back to the starting position. Repeat this movement with one leg and then the other. (See page 142.)

3. Lower one leg slightly to the floor, and then bring it back to the starting position. Repeat with your other leg.

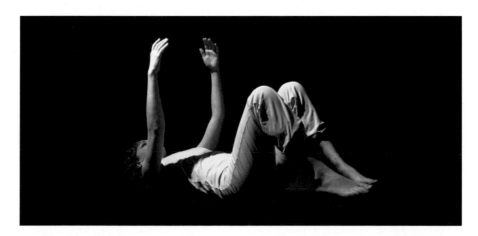

Exercise 10: The Little Airplane

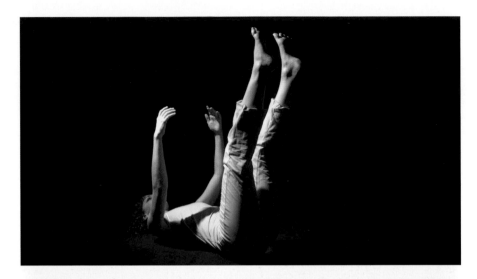

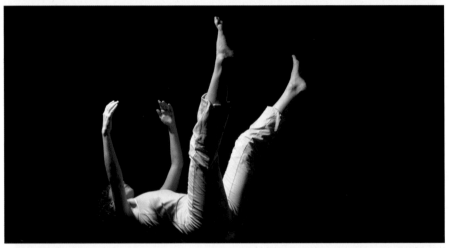

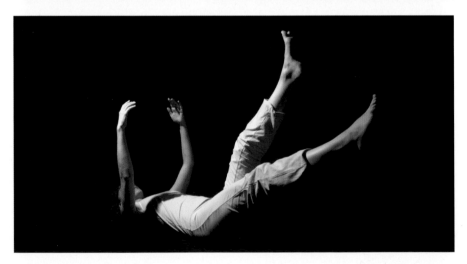

Coordinate the Abdominals

4. Perform the arm stretch (step 1) with one arm and the leg stretch (step 2) with the leg on the opposite side of the body. Bring them back to the starting position and then repeat with the opposite arm and leg.

5. Extend both arms straight up, then drop them together slightly to one side. Return to center.

"Landing"

Separate your legs a little. Start to lower your legs toward the floor. Try to balance laterally on the ball and keep your pelvis from going into anteversion as you continue to slowly lower your legs. The goal is to place both of your feet on the floor at the same time.

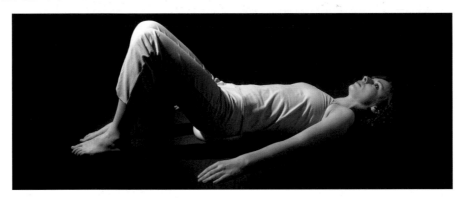

This exercise has several benefits:

- It works the abdominals intensely without placing pressure on either the perineum or the abdominal walls.
- It alternates contractions of the broad muscles among each other and with the rectus abdominis.

Important Note

Exercise 10, "The Little Airplane," is contraindicated for persons with certain conditions:

- It flattens the lower back, eliminating the lordotic curve, so it is not recommended for persons with certain lower back problems.
- It places the pelvis higher than the trunk, sending the abdominal mass and the blood toward the heart. Like all inverted postures, it is not recommended for those with cardiac problems or high blood pressure.

Exercise 10: The Little Airplane

The Drawback Lunge

Exercise 11

Stretching the Rectus Abdominis
with the Drawback Lunge

Stand with your feet parallel and your arms at your sides.

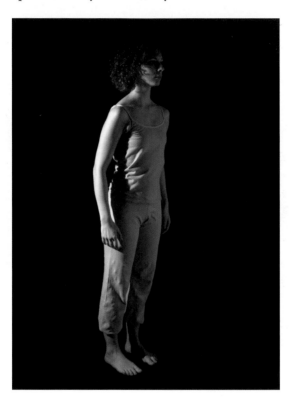

Use Arm Movements to Stretch the
Rectus Abdominis ("Lengthen")

1. Stretch both arms toward the ceiling at the same time, crossing your hands and reaching up as far as possible.
2. Feel how this movement lifts the ribs and stretches the upper region of the rectus abdominis.
3. Return to the starting position.
4. Inhaling deeply into the ribs, repeat this movement, allowing the sternum to lift.
5. Return to starting position.

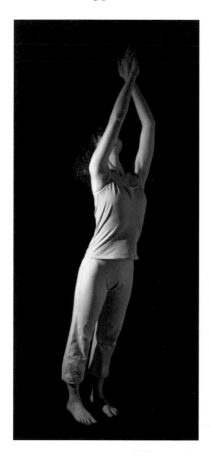 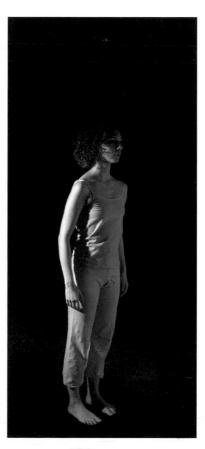

Exercise 11: Stretching the Rectus Abdominis with the Drawback Lunge

Use Leg Movements to Stretch the
Rectus Abdominis ("Foot to the Back")

1. Shift your weight to your left leg. Bend your left knee and, at the same time, extend your right leg behind you as far as possible.
2. Feel how the right side of the pelvis tilts into anteversion. Allow this to happen, and feel how this movement stretches the lower region of the rectus abdominis.
3. Return to the starting position.
4. Inhaling deeply into the ribs, repeat this movement.
5. Return to the starting position.

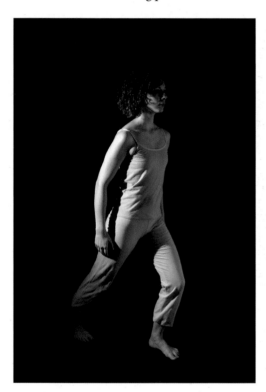 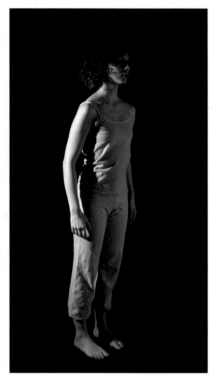

The Drawback Lunge

Use Arm and Leg Movements to Stretch the
Rectus Abdominis ("Deep Lunge")

1. Perform the "Lengthen" and "Foot to the Back" movements of exercise 11 at the same time.
2. Feel how the whole rectus abdominis is stretched.
3. Return to the starting position.
4. Inhaling deeply into the ribs, repeat this movement, allowing the sternum to lift.
5. Return to the starting position.

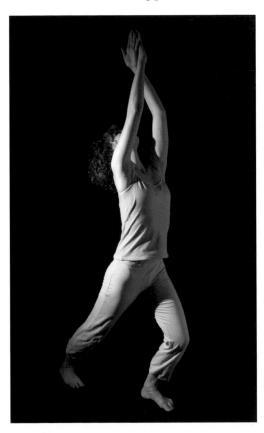 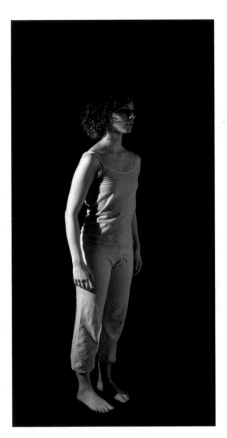

Repeat the Drawback Lunge on the Opposite Side

With your weight on your right leg, extend your left leg behind you as far as possible. In this position, repeat the "Foot to the Back" and the "Deep Lunge" parts of the exercise.

Exercise 11: Stretching the Rectus Abdominis with the Drawback Lunge

Exercise 12

Contracting the Rectus Abdominis with the Drawback Lunge

Contract the Rectus Abdominis in
"Visceral" Mode ("Pull In")

1. With your right leg stretching back and your left leg lunging forward, get into the stretched position of the "Deep Lunge" described in exercise 11.

2. Exhaling, contract the rectus abdominis as if you were trying to bring the pubic bone toward the sternum. Don't allow the exhalation to initiate the movement or lower the ribs. The belly will pull in and the pressure on the perineum will decrease.

3. Return to the starting position.

4. Perform the same movement with your left leg stretching back and your right leg lunging forward.

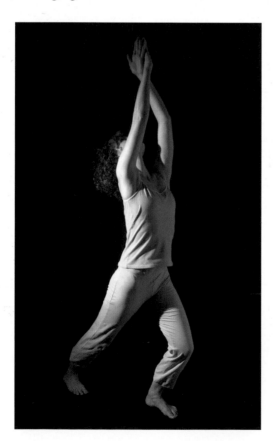 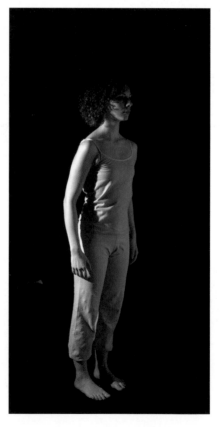

The Drawback Lunge

Contract the Rectus Abdominis in "Skeletal" Mode ("Knee/Hand")

1. Return to the stretched position of the "Deep Lunge" part of exercise 11.
2. Shift your weight to your left leg. Inhaling deeply into your ribs, straighten your left leg, and bend your right leg and sweep it to the front of your body. At the same time, bring your hands down, setting your left hand on your right knee and pushing downward, as if you were trying to push the leg back to the floor. Resist the push, keeping your leg up.

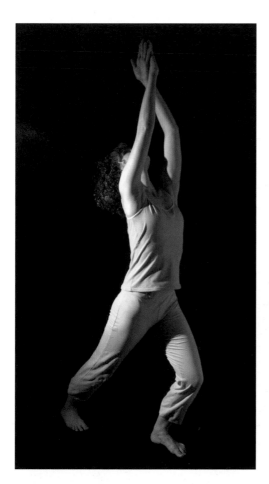
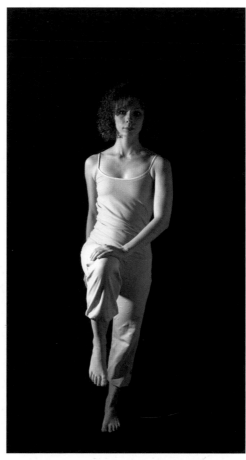

Exercise 12: Contracting the Rectus Abdominis with the Drawback Lunge

3. Exhaling, bring your right leg back to the floor behind you, and then return to the starting position.
4. Inhaling into your ribs, repeat the movement.
5. Exhaling, return to starting position.
6. Perform the same movement on the other side.
7. Relax as you breath normally.
8. Repeat the series one more time.

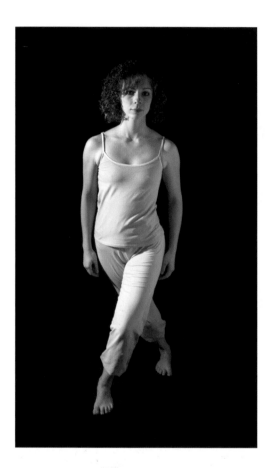 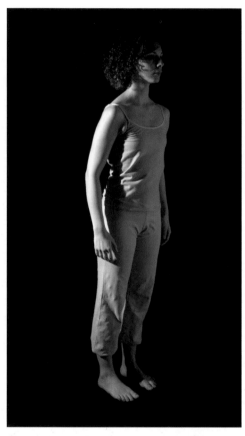

The Drawback Lunge

The Turning Lunge

Exercise 13

Stretching the Obliques with the Turning Lunge

Stand with your feet parallel and your arms at your sides.

Use Arm Movement to Stretch the Internal Obliques ("Lengthen")

1. Bring your right arm up, reaching overhead to the left, stretching as far as possible.
2. Feel how this movement lifts the ribs and stretches the upper region of the right internal oblique.
3. Return to starting position.
4. Inhaling deeply into the ribs, repeat this movement, letting the ribs rise.
5. Return to the starting position.

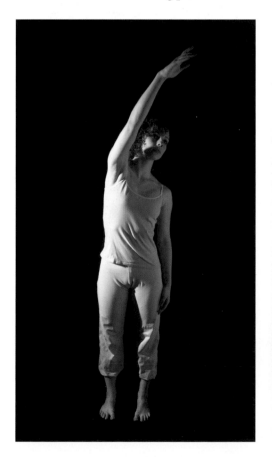 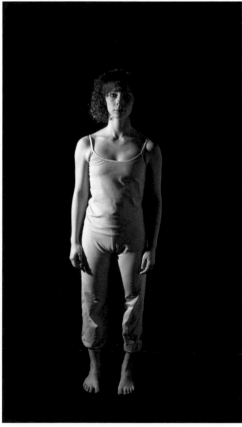

Exercise 13: Stretching the Obliques with the Turning Lunge

Use Leg Movement to Stretch the Internal Obliques
("Foot Crossed")

1. Shift your weight to your left leg. Bend your left knee and, at the same time, extend your right leg behind you, crossing it behind the left leg as far as possible.
2. Feel how the right side of your pelvis turns to the back. Just allow this rotation to happen. This movement stretches the lower region of the right internal oblique.
3. Return to the starting position.
4. Inhaling deeply into the ribs, repeat this movement.
5. Return to the starting position.

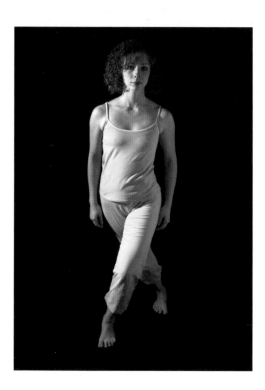 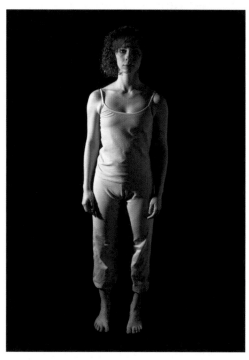

The Turning Lunge

Use Arm and Leg Movements to Stretch the Internal Obliques
("Extreme Lunge")

1. Perform the "Lengthen" and "Foot Crossed" movements of exercise 13 at the same time.
2. Feel how this movement stretches the entire internal oblique.
3. Return to the starting position.
4. Inhaling deeply into the ribs, repeat this movement, letting the ribs rise up.
5. Return to the starting position.

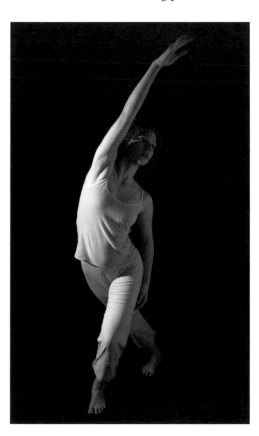 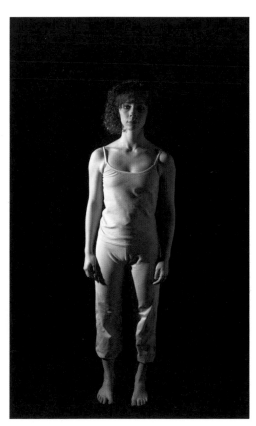

Repeat the Turning Lunge on the Other Side

1. Repeat the "Lengthen" part of the exercise using your left arm.
2. Repeat the "Foot Crossed" part of the exercise with your left leg extended and crossed behind you.
3. Repeat the "Extreme Lunge" part of the exercise with your left arm and leg extended.

Exercise 13: Stretching the Obliques with the Turning Lunge

Exercise 14

Contracting the Obliques with the Turning Lunge

Contract the Abdominals in "Visceral" Mode ("Pull In")

1. Take up the "Extreme Lunge" position of exercise 13.
2. Exhaling, contract your abdominals as if you were trying to bring your pubic bone to your sternum. Don't allow the exhalation to initiate the movement or lower the ribs. The belly will pull in and the pressure on the perineum will decrease.
3. Return to the starting position.

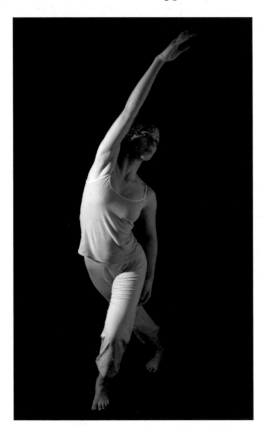 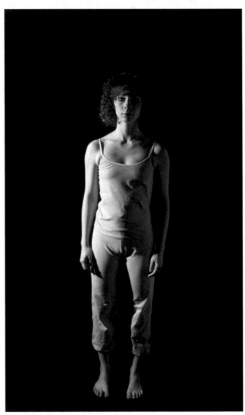

Contract the Right Internal Oblique in "Skeletal" Mode ("Knee/Hand")

1. Perform the "Pull In" movement of exercise 14, as described above, in step 2.
2. Shift your weight to your left leg. Inhaling deeply into your ribs, straighten your left leg, and bend your right leg and sweep it to the front of your body. At the same time, bring your hands down, setting your left hand on your right knee and

pushing downward, as if you were trying to push the leg back to the floor. Resist the push, keeping your leg up.

3. Exhaling, return to the starting position.
4. Perform the movement on the other side.
5. Relax as you inhale and exhale normally.
6. Repeat the series one more time.

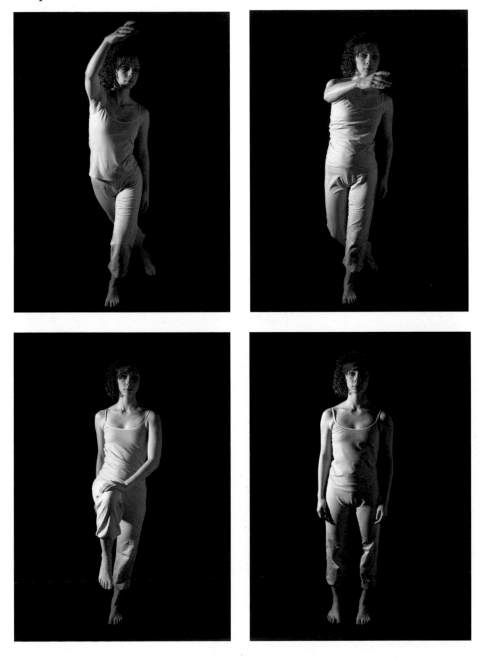

Exercise 14: Contracting the Obliques with the Turning Lunge

The Side Lunge

Exercise 15

Stretching the Obliques with the Side Lunge

Stand with your feet parallel and your arms at your sides.

Use Arm Movement to Stretch the Right Oblique ("Lengthen")

1. Bring your right arm up toward the ceiling. Trace a large arc above your head, letting the weight of the arm bend your trunk to the left.
2. Feel how this movement lifts the right ribs and stretches the upper obliques between the ribs and the pelvis.
3. Return to the starting position.
4. Inhaling deeply into the ribs, perform the movement again, letting the ribs rise.
5. Return to the starting position.

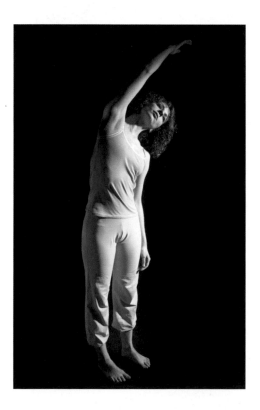 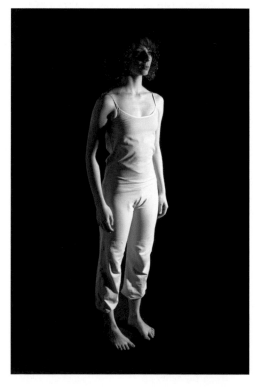

Use the Opposite Arm and Leg
to Stretch the Obliques ("Extreme Lunge")

1. Shift your weight onto your left leg, bending it slightly, and stretch your right leg out to the side.

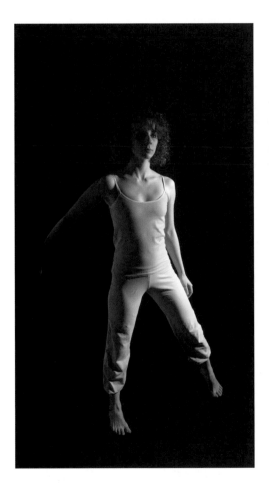 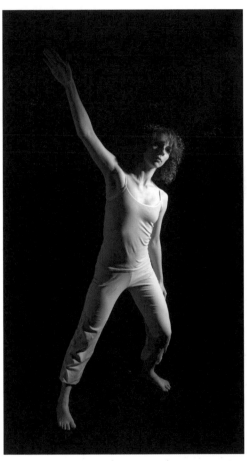

2. In this position, repeat the "Lengthen" movement described in the preceding section of exercise 15.

3. This position allows you to laterally flex the trunk a bit more. Feel how this has the benefit of stretching the obliques.

4. Return to the starting position.

5. Inhaling deeply into the ribs, perform the same movement.

6. Return to the starting position.

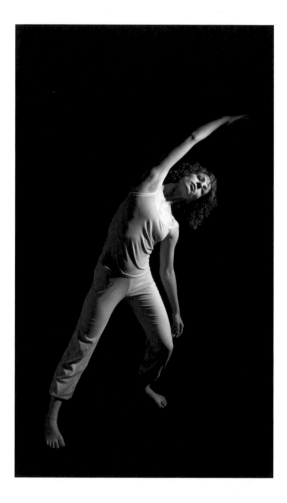 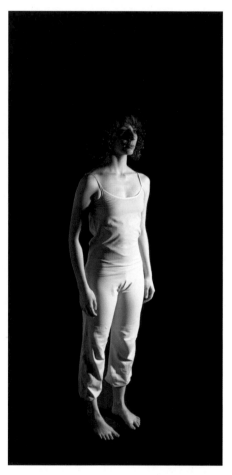

Repeat the Side Lunge on the Opposite Side

1. Repeat the "Lengthen" part of the exercise using your left arm.

2. Repeat the "Extreme Lunge" part of the exercise with your weight on your right leg and your left arm stretching up and over.

The Side Lunge

Exercise 16

Contracting the Obliques with the Side Lunge

Stand with your feet parallel and your arms at your sides.

*Contract the Obliques in "Visceral" Mode
("Pull In")*

1. Take up the "Extreme Lunge" position of exercise 15.
2. Exhaling, contract the abdominals as if you were trying to bring the pubic bone to the sternum and the right ribs toward the pelvis. Don't allow the exhalation to initiate the movement or lower the ribs. The belly will pull in and the pressure on the perineum will decrease.
3. Return to the starting position.
4. Repeat on the other side.

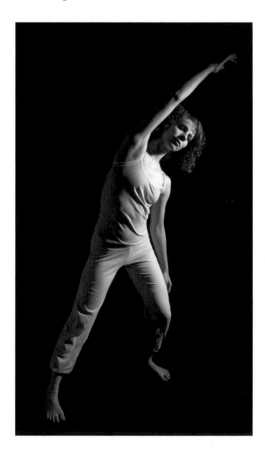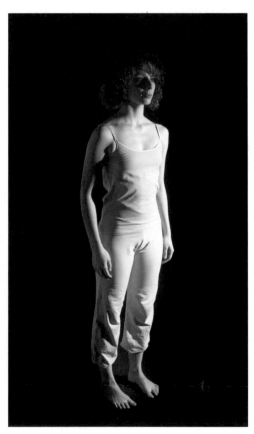

Use Leg Movement to Contract
the Rectus Abdominis ("Knee/Hand")

1. Take up the "Pull In" stretch of exercise 16, as described above.
2. Shift your weight to your left leg. Inhaling deeply into your ribs, straighten your left leg, and bend your right leg and sweep it to the front of your body. At the same time, bring your hands down, setting your left hand on your right knee and

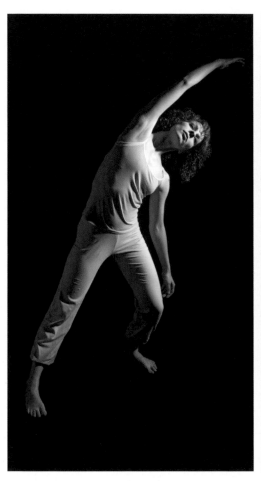 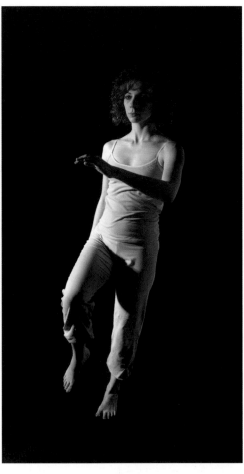

The Side Lunge

pushing downward, as if you were trying to push the leg back to the floor. Resist the push, keeping your leg up.

3. Exhaling, return to the starting position.
4. Perform the movement on the other side.
5. Relax as you inhale and exhale normally.
6. Repeat the series one more time.

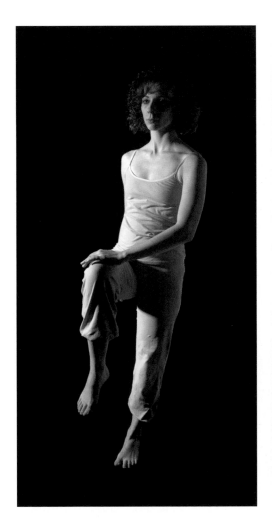 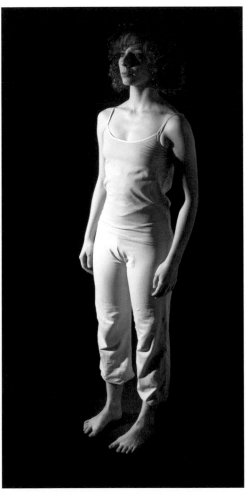

Exercise 16: Contracting the Obliques with the Side Lunge

IMPORTANT IDEAS TO REMEMBER

ABDOMINAL EXERCISES AND A FLAT BELLY: THE TRUTH

The abdominals don't always flatten the belly.

Certain abdominal exercises cause the abdominals to bulge out (pages 41–42).

We can very easily pull in the belly without contracting the abdominals (page 42).

Certain abdominal muscles narrow the waist but don't flatten the belly (pages 42–43).

It's not beneficial to always keep the belly flat (page 43).

The abdominals aren't the only factor to consider if you want a flat belly (pages 45–48).

To have a flat belly, you need to work the abdominals in a specific way (pages 49–54).

THE INHERENT RISKS IN ABDOMINAL EXERCISES

Risks for the perineum (pages 65, 81–82, and 90)

Risks for the abdominal wall (pages 62–63)

Risks for the intervertebral disks and the back (pages 66–67, 69, 78, 82, and 86)

Risks for the cervical disks (pages 70–71)

USER'S GUIDE FOR A FLAT BELLY

Alternately stretch and contract the abdominals (page 49).

Alternately contract the broad muscles (pages 50–51).

Alternately contract the broad muscles and the rectus abdominis (page 51).

Coordinate the contraction of the abdominals with one another (page 52).

Coordinate the contraction of the abdominals with the breath (page 53).

COURSES IN THE "NO-RISK ABS" METHOD

If you wish to find a course that uses the No-Risk Abs techniques, go to our website to find a list of qualified instructors: **www.calais-germain.com**.

Deepen Your Knowledge

Our thirty-hour workshops allow you to expand your knowledge of the abdominals and abdominal exercise. The topics covered include:

- Anatomy of the abdominals
- The action of each muscle on the bones and on the abdomen
- Analysis of the classical abdominal exercises
- Abdominals and their relation to the back muscles
- Abdominals and breathing
- Abdominals and the perineum
- Initial exercises in the No-Risk Abs method
- Avoiding injury

Teaching the No-Risk Abs Method

Our sixty-hour course qualifies you to teach the method to others.

Practice

Complete repertoire of exercises

- Floor work
- Standing work
- Seated work
- Four-point work

Anatomical analysis of each exercise

Pedagogical analysis of each exercise

Breathing patterns

Special cases

Transitions for different levels of practice

Theory

Materials covering anatomy of the viscera and spine

Sequencing of exercises for various levels of practice

Materials covering pathologies commonly found in participants of group classes

Exercises for specific pathologies

Testing Procedures

Written test

Critiqued teaching of a group class

Oral test on theory

Upon completion of training, you have the option of receiving a certificate of completion that allows you to teach the No-Risk Abs Method.

FURTHER READING

Books by Blandine Calais-Germain

Anatomy of Breathing. Seattle: Eastland Press, 2006.

Anatomy of Movement. Rev. ed. Seattle: Eastland Press, 2007.

Anatomy of Movement: Exercises (with Andrée Lamotte). Seattle: Eastland Press, 2008.

The Female Pelvis: Anatomy & Exercises. Seattle: Eastland Press, 2003.

Recommended Reading

Clemente, Carmine D. *Anatomy: A Regional Atlas of the Human Body.* 6th ed. Philadelphia: Lippincott Williams & Wilkins, 2010.

Dolto, Boris. *Le corps entre les mains* [Your body and your hands]. Paris: Vuibert, 2006.

Kapandji, I. A. *The Physiology of the Joints.* 3 vols. 6th ed. London: Churchill Livingstone, 2007 and 2008.

Kendall, H. O., F. P. Kendall, and G. E. Wadsworth. *Muscles: Testing and Function.* 2nd. ed. Baltimore: Williams & Wilkins, 1971.

Marieb, Elaine N., and Katja Hoehn. *Human Anatomy & Physiology.* 8th ed. San Francisco: Benjamin Cummings/Pearson Education, 2009.

Netter, Frank H. *Atlas of Human Anatomy.* 5th ed. Philadelphia: Saunders/Elsevier, 2011.

Rouvière, Henri, and A. Delmas. *Anatomie humaine descriptive et topographique* [Topographical and descriptive human anatomy]. 3 vols. Paris: Masson, 1985.

Vigué-Martin. *Atlas of the Human Body.* Surrey, UK: Rebo International BV, 2005.

INDEX

Page numbers in *italics* refer to illustrations.

BOOKS OF RELATED INTEREST

No-Risk Pilates
8 Techniques for a Safe Full-Body Workout
by Blandine Calais-Germain and Bertrand Raison

The New Rules of Posture
How to Sit, Stand, and Move in the Modern World
by Mary Bond

Pilates on the Ball
A Comprehensive Book and DVD Workout
by Colleen Craig

The Therapeutic Yoga Kit
Sixteen Postures for Self-Healing
through Quiet Yin Awareness
by Cheri Clampett and Biff Mithoefer

The Yin Yoga Kit
The Practice of Quiet Power
by Biff Mithoefer

The Heart of Yoga
Developing a Personal Practice
by T. K. V. Desikachar

The Five Tibetans
Five Dynamic Exercises for Health,
Energy, and Personal Power
by Christopher S. Kilham

Acupressure Taping
The Practice of Acutaping for Chronic Pain and Injuries
by Hans-Ulrich Hecker, M.D., and Kay Liebchen, M.D.

Inner Traditions • Bear & Company
P.O. Box 388
Rochester, VT 05767
1-800-246-8648
www.InnerTraditions.com

Or contact your local bookseller